More Praise ~~for~~ Getting Whole, Getting Well

"*Getting Whole, Getting Well* offers a steady compass for the complex path of chronic illness. These are the very concepts transforming the practice of medicine. Physicians and healers will use this book to inform and inspire their own patients. A tremendous comfort for both individuals and their families. Truly a personal road map to lasting wellness."

Rosa N. Schnyer, LAc, Author of *Acupuncture in the Treatment of Depression* and *Curing Depression Naturally with Chinese Medicine*

"Dr. Iris Bell's *Getting Whole, Getting Well* is a wonderfully practical book full of deep wisdom. She differentiates treatments and therapies that provide real healing as distinct from those that tend to simply suppress disease or temporarily get rid of symptoms. Reading this book is itself healing."

Dana Ullman, MPH, Author of *The Homeopathic Revolution: Why Famous People and Cultural Heroes Choose Homeopathy* and founder of www.homeopathic.com

"*Getting Whole, Getting Well* is a truly great book. Dr. Bell has a knack for putting together seemingly stray bits of information in a practical, meaningful, and even inspiring way, to help you with your own health challenges. This book transcends the "it is your fault that you are ill" attitude that is otherwise common in some forms of conventional and alternative medicine. In reality, you are your own decision maker; and new approaches can turn around the course of your illness toward improved health."

Doris J. Rapp, MD, Author of *Our Toxic World, A Wake Up Call*, www.drrapp.com

GETTING WHOLE, GETTING WELL

ALSO BY DR. IRIS BELL

Clinical Ecology: A New Medical Approach to Environmental Illness

Chew on Things – It Helps You Think: Words of Wisdom from a Worried Canine

Chew on Things Workbook for Fellow Worriers

GETTING WHOLE, GETTING WELL

Healing Holistically from Chronic Illness

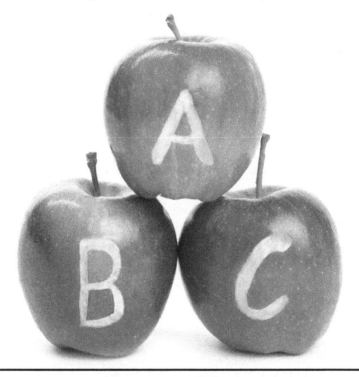

Iris R. Bell, MD PhD

NEW YORK

GETTING WHOLE, GETTING WELL

By Iris R. Bell, MD PhD

ISBN: 978-1-60037-387-9   Paperback

Library of Congress Control Number: 2008920323

Published by:

MORGAN · JAMES
THE ENTREPRENEURIAL PUBLISHER™

Morgan James Publishing, LLC
1225 Franklin Ave Ste 325
Garden City, NY 11530-1693
Toll Free 800-485-4943
www.MorganJamesPublishing.com

Cover and Interior Design by:

Heather Kirk
www.GraphicsByHeather.com
Heather@GraphicsByHeather.com

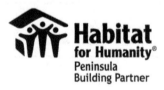

Habitat
for Humanity®
Peninsula
Building Partner

Disclaimer/
Legal Notice

This document is intended to provide general educational information regarding the subject matter covered. It is not intended to provide specific or personalized medical advice or treatment, and the reader is advised to seek and obtain specific and personalized medical advice and treatment from his or her own qualified health care providers. Neither the author nor the publisher assumes any responsibility for any errors or omissions. The author and publisher also specifically disclaim any responsibility or liability resulting from the use of the information and suggestions given in this book or from the use of websites, books, audiovisual products, biofeedback equipment, or other resources listed in this document.

The information provided here offers an educational resource and is not intended to serve as medical advice related to any person's specific health problems. There can be no assurance that any person's specific health problems, diseases, or symptoms will heal, recover, or otherwise resolve as a result of applying the information provided in this document or through any other documents, audiofiles, or other media obtained from the Resources list. There also can be no assurance of safety with or absence of possible harm from any specific treatment or therapy if a specific person tries such treatment or therapy mentioned in this document or in any other documents, audiofiles, or other media obtained from the Resources list.

To everyday miracles for us all.

Contents

Acknowledgments

In Latin, the word "doctor" means" teacher." In reality, we are all teachers for each other, whether or not anointed with a formal degree. My own education in illness, health, health care and healing has come from many different doctors, nurses, healers, and other health care providers, official and unofficial teachers (including numerous practitioners of various healing professions, patients, friends, colleagues, and strangers), and personal inner experiences.

With that definition, I would say that some of my teachers enraged me; some supported and nurtured me; and some don't even know me. All of them led me to think and feel - and learn. The list of my real teachers is too long to fit into this book without boring everyone whose name does not appear and annoying anyone whose name I forget. A special thanks to my father, who told me not to let contradictions throw me. He said they'd be everywhere, and he was right.

I learn daily from a myriad of people and sources, sometimes in a slowly dawning realization over many years, sometimes in a flash of surprising insight in a moment. Healing seems to be so much a lifelong journey, and all healing is truly self-healing. To each person who has helped teach me along my own journey, thank you for your wisdom, intentional or otherwise. As Mark van Doren, the American educator and writer said, "The art of teaching is the art of assisting discovery." And, for me, discovery is the essence of life.

Foreword

From the national evening news, blaring on the front pages of major newspapers, to internet websites and blogs, we are deluged by the panacea of the moment, with claims from both conventional and alternative medicine. Conflicting scientific outcomes are bewildering, life threatening pharmaceutical recalls abound, and today's miracle cure becomes tomorrow's nightmare.

How does an individual know what to select or, even more demanding, how to combine the best of conventional and alternative interventions into an "integrative medicine" approach that insures the best outcomes for both patient and practitioner? Fortunately, this dilemma is addressed and resolved by Dr. Iris Bell through her *Getting Whole, Getting Well* program.

Having known and worked with Dr. Bell as a colleague and friend for over 30 years, she is literally the best person to help all of us sort out this bewildering array of options. When I have had a question in such matters or how to interpret the results of a complex research study, I have always relied on the honesty, integrity, excellent scientific and clinical skills, as well as the compassion of Dr. Bell.

Trained as a conventional physician and now a Professor of Family and Community Medicine at the University of Arizona College of Medicine, she is truly a world-class expert with a loving heart and deeply spiritual orientation. Gandhi exhorted his followers to "Be the change you wish to see manifest in the world" and that is Dr Bell's philosophy as well.

Bits and pieces of what to do abound, but what is needed is an overall plan or strategy to make sense of these disparate parts. Any effective treatment plan involves conventional and alternative medicine, self care practices, different clinicians and practitioners, as well as an abiding personal tenacity or "will to live" to achieve optimal health and well being.

Getting Whole, Getting Well provides this map to integrate, coordinate and organize this multifaceted approach. Based on the **"ABC Principle,"** Dr. Bell details her three steps of: 1) **Assess** — to know your full array of options; 2) **Balance** — know that you are a living, dynamic being and how to balance all the treatments; and, 3) **Coordinate** — Make connections between your practices and practitioners rather than a patchwork of disconnected pieces. Through this ABC approach, Dr. Bell provides a clean and practical approach born out of her decades of clinical practice, research, and personal experience.

"Physis" is the Latin root of the word physician, and it has both an external and internal dimension. Externally, the role of the healer was to harmonize the individual with his or her physical, social and cultural environment. Internally, "physis" referred to the "healing force within." Today, as in the roots of all healing traditions, the role of the physician and healer is to harmonize the individual with the environment and elicit the healing forces within. It is in keeping with this perennial wisdom and timeless compassion that Dr. Bell provides all of us with a practical, effective, and compassionate map of our unique pathway to optimal health and well being.

Kenneth R. Pelletier, PhD, MD(hc)
Clinical Professor of Medicine
University of Arizona College of Medicine
    and University of California School of Medicine
    (UCSF) San Francisco
Author of *New Medicine: Family Health Guide*

Introduction

Learn the Big Picture of Chronic Disease and Health Care: The ABC Principle for Your Personalized Holistic Healing

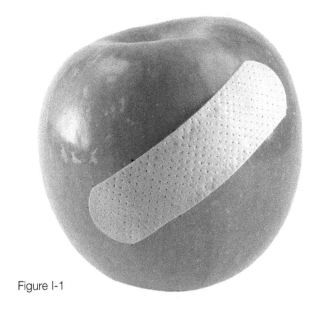

Figure I-1

"It's no longer a question of staying healthy. It's a question of finding a sickness you like."
~Jackie Mason

The Bad — *The Problem of Chronic Conditions*

In the past century, chronic diseases (those lasting 6 months or more) such as heart disease, stroke, diabetes, cancer, lung diseases, arthritis, and many others have become a much larger health problem in the U.S. and other developed nations than are infectious diseases. One out of every ten Americans suffers from a chronic disabling condition such as arthritis, back problems, a heart or lung condition that reduces quality of life over periods of years. Seventy percent of the deaths in the U.S. each year are due to a chronic disease. Seventy-eight percent of health care costs are for treatment of chronic diseases. In short, chronic disease eventually touches all of us -- ourselves and our families.

The Ugly — *The Risks and Confusion of Current Health Care*

"His sickness increases from the remedies applied to cure it."
~Virgil

Although modern mainstream medicine has made many amazing advances in prolonging lives and controlling symptoms, people with chronic diseases know from their own experience that the available treatments often bring many limitations, side effects, and problems. For example, a study published in the *Journal of the American Medical Association* estimated that over 2 million hospitalized patients in 1994 experienced adverse drug reactions, including over 100,000 fatal drug reactions.

The number of deaths from "properly" prescribed drugs placed prescription drugs as the sixth leading cause of death in this country, after heart disease, cancer, stroke, lung disease, and accidents and before pneumonia and diabetes. Yet, eighty percent of older adults take at least three medications daily. Patients on five drugs also have a 50-50 risk of suffering from an adverse drug interaction. The rates of adverse reactions seem to be rising even more in recent follow-up studies.

Meanwhile, persons with and without chronic diseases seek out complementary and alternative medicine **(CAM)** of various types in large numbers — including prayer — 75% of American adults have used CAM, most often for pain problems in the back, neck, and joints. For many chronic diseases, the majority of affected persons use both conventional and CAM treatments. They usually do not even inform their physician that they are doing so. At the same time, health care providers are recognizing more and more adverse interactions between drugs (both prescription and non-prescription types) and natural products such as herbs.

Conventional medical care and patients are at a crisis point – high costs, low patient and provider satisfaction with the health care process, many confusing options, and a growing chronic disease burden on society and the individual. How does a person with chronic disease find a way out of this box?

This book is intended for people with chronic illnesses of all types who prefer to have a big picture plan or roadmap of strategy and tactics before diving into the specifics of dealing with any life challenge — in health or another area.

The Good — *The Option of Personalized Holistic Healing with the ABC Principle*

The point of the book is that you can learn to build your own effective individualized program of holistic healing care that includes practitioner-provided and self-care interventions – but you have to understand where each option fits into the big picture. Most other books on CAM are either introductory overview encyclopedias of treatment modalities or in depth explanations of one type of CAM. But, all CAM treatments — just as with Western medicine — are not the same, in terms of their potential to help different people with different types of health conditions.

As a consumer, you probably find it hard to decide what is best for you. Many people combine treatments without giving much thought to interactions — good or bad — between them, let alone the potential for the package of care to help them overall.

Picking treatments just because you prefer something more familiar or easier to do, rather than something less familiar and harder to try could keep you from maximizing your results. And, picking treatments — or, sometimes, providers, because they helped Aunt Alma is no guarantee that you'll get what you need to solve your problems. For many people with chronic illnesses, putting together a handful of vitamins and minerals and herbs is a way to start, but it is usually not enough. True healing is a complex but rewarding journey, not an overnight cure from a magic pill. Putting your options into a larger perspective will make it much clearer for you to know what to do.

This book is different. *Getting Whole, Getting Well* gives you an alternative to the confusion — with the ABC Principle of personalized holistic healing. The ABC Principle is a way to create your own individualized plan for getting the most benefit and least risk from the integrated package of care that you will develop. Throughout this book, you will see these ideas at work:

Assess

Assess your options and how they might help you. Re-assess the benefits and risks before you begin and periodically throughout treatment for each intervention and for the package of care that you choose

Balance

Balance yourself as a living system whose body parts all play different, essential, and interrelated roles within you, by balancing the elements of your treatment package to serve your ability as a whole not only to survive, but also to thrive

Coordinate

Coordinate the elements of your treatment plan as a whole, interconnected system of care intended to balance you, not as a patchwork collection of things-I'd-like-to-try-and-see-what-helps-each-separate-symptom

The word "holistic" is seemingly out of fashion. People talk instead, more recently, about "complementary and alternative medicine" and "integrative medicine" as a way of explaining the political role of certain treatments within the larger health care system, where conventional Western medicine is assumed to be "best." But Western medicine treats a person as a patchwork collection of body parts, each treated ("fixed") separately. A major limitation of emphasizing the name for the treatment type is that we lose sight of the main point. That is, any treatment is in the service of the person who wants and needs to heal as a whole being.

A person does not seek help to heal by using a specific treatment tool. "Holistic" brings the focus back onto the person, where it belongs. The underlying message is the importance of the holistic, systemic nature of the person, the goal of balance among the person's interconnected and indivisible "parts" (whether labeled by Western medicine or by CAM with different diagnoses or words), and the facilitating role for a coordinated package of care in helping the person achieve balance.

Many forms of CAM diagnose a person in an individualized way. But, the process of true holism involves more than honoring a person's preferences. True holism is also more than acknowledging spiritual, mental, emotional, social, and physical aspects of a person as if each of these aspects were a body part to treat separately. The truly holistic use of CAM inherently coordinates the elements of care toward the singular goal of balancing and healing the whole person as a unique individual...that is, Personalized Holistic Healing.

Critics point out that conventional Western medicine often emphasizes the diagnosis (disease-centered care) rather than the person with the condition (person-centered care). By our choice of language, we have made a subtle shift away from recognition that it is the person who has whatever manifestations of illness he or she experiences. Our language instead labels us as being the manifestations, the symptoms, the diagnosis. It is time to think about symptoms and conditions as clues to a fundamental imbalance present throughout the person, an imbalance that holistic treatment can gently set back into balance and then maintain. Then the person will manifest wellness.

The material here offers my own personal and professional perspective, based on over 30 years of being both a patient and a professional with one foot in mainstream medicine and the other in alternative medicine. I have learned that there are answers for each of us, but no simple prescription is good for everyone. So, to each person on his or her journey of healing — Godspeed to you.

Iris R. Bell, MD PhD
ibell@GettingWhole.com • www.IrisBell.com
Tucson, Arizona

Chapter 1

Start on the Healing Road – Again and Always, Ready or Not

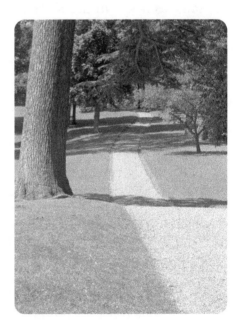

Figure 1-1

"Toto — I've a feeling we're not in Kansas anymore."
~Dorothy in *The Wizard of Oz*

One of my favorite movies is the *Wizard of Oz*. In telling its timeless and entertaining story, the movie teaches many essential life lessons. It is the story of a young girl from a Kansas farm, Dorothy Gale, whose world gets turned upside down and transported over the rainbow by what she experiences as a tornado. Everything she believed, thought, and did in her usual world is different. Scarecrows talk, trees come alive and throw apples, monkeys fly, witches pop in and out — nothing is the same as it was in her Kansas world.

People with chronic illnesses find themselves shocked and bewildered when they are displaced from "normal" everyday life into their own new world of difficulties. Your usual life has been swept away by your own personal tornado and dumped into an unknown land with unknown people and new rules about how things work. Not only do you have to deal with figuring out how to get the best health care, but you also have to adjust your goals, dreams, relationships, and everyday life around your illness. How you deal with the difficulties determines how your story ends.

This book gives you a way to look at the process of having one or more chronic diseases and of healing yourself as the individual who experiences them. This is not a one-minute solution to chronic illness or an ordinary list of how-to's and where to get help. It is a practical health philosophy book for people who need to make sense of what has happened to them. The book helps you see your illness pattern in a larger context and to discern how to select from and orchestrate the overwhelming options for treatment that bombard you with promises of cure.

"Pay no…attention to that man behind the curtain."
~The Wizard of Oz

Some people quit and let the disease take over. They go to sleep in the poppy field and don't wake up. Some find ways to cope and accept their limitations. They may find their way to Oz, but they never leave — they just proceed to live in their bearable, but stuck place. And some seek ways to "fix" the problem. Those people try to find the Wizard of Oz, who, they expect, has "The Answer" for making the problem miraculously go away. The thing is, the Wizard is often, at best, a well-intentioned caring mortal who really can't change their problem very much, or at worst, a fraud who makes promises he cannot keep.

You are a unique individual who needs a unique package of care and tailored advice. You must develop a self-directed plan for choosing the healing mentors and using the package of healing methods best for you. You will go through a great deal to learn that you have gathered the answers all along the way — so that, in the end, you are ready to click your heels and say, "There's no place like home, there's no place like home, there's no place like home." And you get home. To health.

But how do you figure out this special plan? It's a secret that only a few people stumble upon in their lives. The secret is that you have to go home to yourself, your true self, by way of your own personal life journey down a yellow brick road of obstacles, mystery, and change. There are both spiritual and practical steps you can and must take to heal.

Health problems are part of your life's journey; they are not detours that take you off your path. You can't force your body to stop having a disease or symptoms. If you do, more problems will pop up somewhere else. Get help staying on the road, assembling tools, supporters and fellow travelers, until the healing happens in its own time, in your own time, with your own answer.

Five personal qualities necessary to carry you through your challenges with chronic illness are:

- Courage (The Cowardly Lion)
- Heart (The Tin Woodman)
- Clarity in thinking (The Scarecrow)
- Persistence (Dorothy)
- Openness to change (Dorothy)

> Glinda, the Good Witch — *"You don't need to be helped any longer. You've always had the power to go back to Kansas."*
>
> Dorothy — *"I have?"*

Scarecrow — *"Then why didn't you tell her before?"*

Glinda, the Good Witch — *"Because she wouldn't have believed me. She had to learn it for herself."*

In addition, you also need the right information, social support (a scarecrow, a lion, a tin woodsman, and a Toto, not to mention Auntie Em and Uncle Henry), and the ability to sort through the information with advice from a mentor who can see the big picture of your particular situation and help you at the right time. You need a Glinda, the Good Witch of the North, a mentor to point you in the right direction and keep you safe when danger lurks.

In the movie, everybody tells Dorothy that the answer lies in following the yellow brick road to the Wizard. That road is far from safe or straight in getting her where she needs to arrive, but it guides her into the experiences she must live through so that she can ultimately get home.

Getting Whole, Getting Well is your first Glinda to start you off along your own personal yellow brick road with a big picture overview of what happens in disease, health, health care, and, ultimately, self-healing. Many books talk about wellness measures such as diet, exercise, and meditation that are basic and valuable for everyone, but usually not enough to move the person with chronic disease into true healing.

I intend *Getting Whole, Getting Well* to help serve as part of your decision-making process in making informed choices about your health care, but it does not replace the advice of — or treatment from — qualified health care professionals. You will need more mentors and more information, so — seek them out. At appropriate places, I will also point out some additional movie metaphors that illustrate other key ideas.

The point of view is my own, based on my personal and professional experiences with, knowledge of, and opinions about disease, health care, and healing. You might agree or disagree. But it will force you to think about your health and health care in a new way. Just looking at these issues can be a start for you in getting whole, getting well now. And if you build your own personal holistic health care plan with a practical map, you will be on your way.

"*Most people have come to prefer certain of life's experiences and deny and reject others, unaware of the value of the hidden things that may come wrapped in plain and even ugly paper. In avoiding all pain and seeking comfort at all costs, we may be left without intimacy or compassion; in rejecting change and risk we often cheat ourselves of the quest; in denying our suffering we may never know our strength or our greatness.*"

Rachel Naomi Remen, MD

"*Health is a state of complete physical, mental and social well-being, and not merely the absence of disease or infirmity.*"

World Health Organization

Chapter 2

You Are Not a Car:
Change Your Mindset, Not Your Oil

The New ABC Perspective of Whole Person Healing:
You are More than the Sum of Your Body Parts

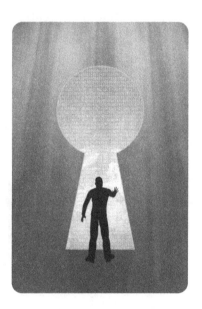

Figure 2-1

"In the book of life, the answers aren't in the back."
~Charlie Brown, *"Peanuts"* comic strip
character created by Charles Schulz

A. Is Your Life a Car or a Hologram?

The trouble is that people with chronic disease have usually accepted the world view of conventional medicine that the body is made of parts that are assembled into some sort of mechanical being. Parts can be removed with surgery or forced to work better with a drug if they malfunction. **To conventional or mainstream medicine, the body is a car whose parts are either unnecessary (appendix, tonsils, gallbladders) or replaceable (hearts, livers, kidneys).** In many emergencies and acute illnesses, the mainstream perspective and treatments can be life-saving. In chronic disease, however, it can lead to problems.

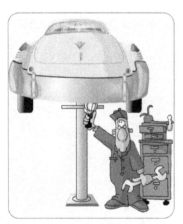

Figure 2-2A
You are not a mechanical object like a car with replaceable body parts.

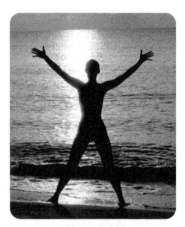

Figure 2-2B
You are a whole indivisible person, a living complex system, an interconnected network unto yourself.

The trouble with the automobile or static mechanical view of the body is that it is incomplete and often wrong. Conventional medicine works best in the short term on local body parts. In the long term, however, a person is a living whole being (in technical terms, an indivisible complex living system), a dynamic (ever-changing) network of inter-related and inseparable parts. The health of any particular part is a reflection of the health of the whole person.

In one sense, a person is more like a hologram than a car. The whole is greater than the sum of the parts, and what each part does at the seemingly local level reflects the condition of the whole person at the global level. A hologram is a three-dimensional image produced by a coherent laser light.

The key feature of a hologram is that any part of a holographic film contains the whole image. Many systems of CAM, including acupuncture and homeopathy, explicitly recognize this holographic reality of the person and use it in their approach to diagnosis and treatment. CAM systems use the local symptoms as a clue to the overall (global) disturbance in the person.

The symptom is a complete, self-contained small picture (microcosm) of the complete big picture (macrocosm) that is the person's disease. CAM treatment ultimately targets the big picture (global) as it reveals itself in the small picture (local) disturbance. Conventional medicine looks at molecules, which are the local level, and stays at the local level to treat the molecular behaviors. The best drugs in conventional medicine target specific cells and molecules, even subtypes of cells and molecules and their receptors in the body at the local level of scale. In contrast, CAM systems use the behaviors of the molecules in order to see the big picture behaviors of the whole system of which the molecules are a part.

Thus, mainstream medicine and systems of CAM approach diagnosis and treatment very differently. As a consumer of health care, you may not realize that you usually apply the much more familiar automobile, local world view of your body when you seek treatment.

In fact, you often use the automobile world view even when you try CAM. You want something to fix the problem you experience in a body part. You usually don't consider that the body part is simply doing its best to tell you that You are sick. Sickness in a body part is a biofeedback message back to you that You are out of balance, out of alignment with your Self and your environment.

The misalignment is not necessarily some conscious decision you made that you can feel guilty over or revisit and do over in a simple way. Rather, the misalignment is a result of the convergence of multiple causes that may range from genetics to lifestyle to environmental stressors and circumstances. Some of the causes are conscious choices you made, but some are very much outside your immediate control.

Your body has a wisdom – it knows that it isn't a car. It knows that it is a hologram. Do you? If you have a symptom – a rash on your skin or a headache or a pain in a joint or diarrhea, you are sick, not your skin or head or joint or gut. It just happens that the only way your skin can manifest your sickness at its own local level is by way of a rash or a pimple.

In short, symptoms are a wake-up call from yourself to Your Self. This is true holistic healing in action. If you can look at your symptoms and diseases in a holographic way, you can come up with remarkable insights and plan your treatment better. Otherwise, every option seems just as good – or bad – as every other option – and there is a bewildering number of options out there from which to choose.

[A reply to letters recommending remedies]:
"Dear Sir (or Madam): I try every remedy sent to me. I am now on No. 67. Yours is 2,653. I am looking forward to its beneficial results."
~Mark Twain quoted in My Father Mark Twain, by Clara Clemens

This book's specific point of view comes from a convergence and an integration of modern thinking in science, *i.e.*, complex systems and network theory, and the ancient wisdom from complementary medicine systems of healing – *i.e.*, classical homeopathy, traditional Chinese medicine, Ayurvedic healing. There is a way to decide which of the 2,653 options make most sense – and how the options you do choose might be best utilized. The rest of this book explains the general principles of how to do so.

B. Zooming your lens up and down the levels of scale in healing.

A person is an intact, indivisible network system. At the same time, a person is part of larger and larger network systems (social groups, the biological, chemical, and physical environment, up to the universe at the highest level) and is comprised of smaller and smaller network systems (organs, cells, molecules). Depending on your perspective, you probably also consider yourself part of an even larger spiritual or transcendent reality. How you view a person or yourself depends on your perspective – that is, if you had a camera that could zoom out to panoramic view or in, down to a microscopic view, you would be able to look at health and disease from different perspectives. The perspectives would be where you stand as the observer.

Regardless of the position of the observer, however, upsetting or perturbing a network system at any level of organization will lead to changes at levels above and below the immediately affected level. That is, a loss or gain of social support from a spouse has an impact, as does exposure to or avoidance of a toxic environmental chemical or a nutritional deficiency or supplement that changes biochemical pathway network function at the molecular level of organization.

Movie Metaphor Moment

In the movie *It's a Wonderful Life*, Jimmy Stewart's character George Bailey hits a low point in his life and contemplates suicide. He feels that he is worth more dead than alive. His angel Clarence lets him experience an alternate reality in which George had never existed, and he learns how important his "meaningless" life has been to many people. If George hadn't been around, his brother Harry would have drowned in childhood by falling through the ice one winter. Then Harry wouldn't have been there to save his fellow soldiers in a World War II battle. George himself wouldn't have been there as an adult with his savings and loan company to save the people in his town from the predatory banker Mr. Potter. The point is that we each have our niche in a much larger network system or universe, and we do not always consciously recognize our role in the big picture. Nevertheless, we are each an essential part of the big picture.

In health care, our usual focus is the person level of organization. In conventional medicine, there is a perspective called "patient-centered care." Patient-centered care, which concerns itself with the issues of who-has-the-disease, is distinguished from disease-centered care, which concerns itself with the issues of what-is-the-disease. **In other words, the person is more important than his/her disease label.**

Disease-centered thinking in conventional medicine revolves around the cellular and molecular level of scale. However, research has shown that many of us prefer to have a relationship with a provider who gives us patient-centered care in the sense that we are informed about our disease(s) and all of our treatment options and participate in decisions about how to proceed (rather than being told what to do).

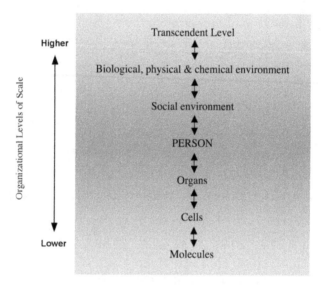

Figure 2-3

Organizational Levels of Scale. You are a system unto yourself, but you are made up of other systems at lower levels of organizational scale (e.g., circulatory system, immune system); and you are a part of still other systems at higher levels of organizational scale (e.g., families, communities, living creatures on earth).

> For a complex living system, each next higher level of organization has emergent properties, that is, behaviors that the higher level can generate, but that its component parts at a lower level cannot (a person has" behaviors" that a liver or heart by itself does not). At the same time, there is a bidirectional feedback loop of information, from the global to the local level and back the other way. It is the feedback that allows the global (person level) and local (body parts level) to influence each other's function, that is, to define your unique "you-ness."

Another way of understanding the holographic qualities of health and healing is to look at levels of scale from a systems perspective – true holism. Many systems, especially living systems, have a self-similarity or theme (also called "fractality"), at every level of scale. The self-similarity is a geometric concept in which an object is irregular but similarly irregular at every degree of magnification, *i.e.*, close up and far away.

One example from nature is a pine tree (see photo series in Figure 2-3A to 2-3C). From forest level of scale to a single tree to a branch with pine cone to close-up detail of a pine cone, the irregular appearances are similar. Look at the pictures – zoom in left to right. Zoom out right to left. You see some similar visual themes in the way the pine forest, individual pine tree, and single pine cone look, whether you zoom in or zoom out as you look at the scene across the set of pictures. One obvious theme, for example, is the irregular pointed tips of each level of organization, with a recurring theme of triangular shapes.

Without question, a forest, a single tree, and a pine cone each has some properties that the other levels of scale in this example do not possess. Nevertheless, some patterns manifest across the different levels of scale.

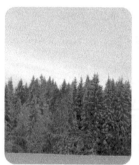
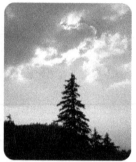
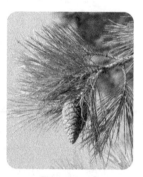

Figure 2-4A	Figure 2-4B	Figure 2-4C
Notice the pattern of the pine forest as a whole – repeated points and triangular shapes across its silhouette	*Notice the pattern of the individual pine tree as a whole – coming to a point and exhibiting triangular shapes throughout its silhouette*	*Notice the pattern of the lone pine cone on the tree – coming to a point at the tip of the triangular shaped pine cone*

In conventional anatomy, the self-similarity occurs in body parts such as different levels of organization of the bronchial tree. In complementary therapies, the self-similarity is not in physical structure so much as it is in patterns of function or dynamics (change). People can be in self-similar ruts of disease, just as they can be in ruts with relationships or jobs. The same idea is true for processes and functions – such as you, your body, and your health in your life.

Thus, under environmental stress (psychological or physical in nature), a person prone to asthma may experience an asthma attack. Their "rut" is responding with anxiety and asthma under certain environmental challenges. A different person might respond to the same environmental factors with irritability and a migraine attack. You are literally "doing your own [unique] thing" in your world. And, in chronic illness, you are doing your own unhealthy thing over and over. The names and faces (specific content or details) may change from event to event, but the storyline repeats the same process through time.

"All change is not growth, as all movement is not forward."
~Ellen Glasgow

C. Life is Dynamical and Non-Linear.

The true nature of living systems is that they are in motion. That is, living systems change all the time. Their pattern of movement through life is nonlinear. That is, small changes on the input side can lead to large changes on the output side.

The resultant changes can be for better or for worse.

For example, an astronaut fires a short burst of a rocket on the space shuttle and thus causes a minor change in the trajectory of the orbit. This small action can tweak the orbit enough to end up sending the shuttle back down to earth... either slowly for a gentle landing with the precisely right rocket firing, or into a devastating ball of fire, with a tiny miscalculation and overshoot.

The nature of the change itself matters to the outcome, as well as the state of the system at the moment the change occurs. In a healthy person without diabetes, a small cut on the foot while running barefoot at the beach (the change) heals without complications in a matter of days. In a diabetic, the same small cut on a foot can expand over days into a raging infection that threatens the leg and ultimately the life of the person. Similarly, it might take hundreds of bee stings from Africanized bees (the change) to put a healthy person into the hospital, whereas one untreated bee sting can kill an allergic person who has bee venom sensitivity on the spot, in a matter of minutes.

At the social level of scale, a seemingly small comment from a friend or a therapist might trigger large changes in another person's behaviors (*e.g.*, stopping addictive use of tobacco or drugs), for example, if the comment arrives at a critical moment in the recipient's life. A seemingly small manipulation of the soft tissue in the back by a massage therapist or insertion of a thin needle at an acupuncture point by an acupuncturist or dissolving a constitutional homeopathic remedy under the tongue can also stimulate a cascade of larger and larger changes that lead to improvements in health far distant across the body-network from the local spot in the body where the treatment was initially applied.

How can such change occur? It happens because of the small-world, perhaps scale-free, network nature of the person as a complex nonlinear dynamical system. **The person really is a whole being who consciously and unconsciously monitors and "cares" about all of his/her parts. The person as a whole and each part "hears about" and reacts to whatever has happened to the whole person or to a part somewhere else in the body.**

Networks involve points of interconnection called nodes. The most highly interconnected nodes are called hubs. In a human being, many whole systems of CAM view the person as an interconnected network of small worlds (local subsystems) that have bridges between the small worlds. The local structure is a mirror of the larger global (whole person) structure. The meridian system of Chinese medicine is one such example of a network viewpoint, in which the nodes are certain acupuncture points along certain meridians that exert greater effects on function.

Sometimes understanding networks is easier when you think about social networks such as a group of friends. Each person has a relationship with every other person in the group, but some are stronger than others. Some individuals emerge as group leaders — their ideas carry more weight with the rest of the members of the group than the opinions of non-leader members.

You may have heard of "six degrees of separation" – that is, social scientists have found that you are within six acquaintances or friends away from contacting anyone else on the planet, famous or unknown, from within your own social network (give or take a couple of people). In fact, people with the weakest links to you, i.e., your acquaintances rather than closest friends, may be the surest way to connect with people outside your immediate social circle. Acquaintances know people that you and your best friends do not (people with strong links to one another tend to know more of the same people) – and so, acquaintances can spread the word for you the best.

In the living person, hubs are like the office water coolers of the body, where information exchange occurs. If you want to hear or spread a rumor, get yourself to the water cooler, where your work acquaintances congregate to catch up on gossip. You will get the information spread wide and far to people whom you yourself do not know very well or at all.

In complex network systems, changes that affect a hub can exert more extensive effects on the rest of the network than do changes affecting a less well-connected node. If the company moves the water cooler to a highly central accessible spot in the office where more people can readily go (making the water cooler an even stronger physical hub for the social network of the office staff), the gossip will spread even more quickly. If the company instead moves the water cooler to a far corner of the building where most people have to walk for a long distance and past the boss's office to get there, the water cooler loses some of its hub status – and gossip spreads more slowly (unless another location in the building takes its place as the popular meeting site on breaks).

A person is an intact, indivisible system unto him or herself as well. Within the person, the body has major hubs such as the brain. The brain controls things that happen in the rest of the body as it evaluates and responds to an endless stream of information from the inner and outer environments. Internally, the information actually flows both ways – from the brain to the rest of the body and vice versa. In general, as a hub, the brain has a bigger influence than do other body parts on how the person behaves in response to changes in the internal and external environments. The body has other important but somewhat less influential hubs, *e.g.*, in the immune system, such as lymph nodes.

Zoom out to the level of society. Network researchers point out, for instance, that in an epidemic disease at the society level of organizational scale, such as HIV/AIDS, treating the hubs (the most sexually active individuals in society) may slow the spread of the infection sooner than treating each isolated case as it arises in persons who are lesser nodes within the social network (sexually less active persons).

Returning to the person level of scale in conventional anatomy, the brain is a major hub, controlling many functions in other parts of the body. A toe is a much less important node at the person level of scale. A person can afford to lose a toe and continue to live with reasonable success in the world, but he/she cannot afford to lose the brain. In acupuncture, the person as a network is made up of meridians (invisible pathways connecting nodes throughout the person) and acupuncture points (certain points are hubs and others are nodes). The electrical properties of the acupuncture points (nodes and hubs) are demonstrably different from those of other points on the skin.

A network implies static structure, but the network also provides the architecture through which information or energy flows in repeated patterns (function). **It is possible for the pattern of the trajectory of the flow in motion to shift.** In chaos theory, a close relative of complexity theory, there are attractors. An attractor is a set of properties to which a system's behavior evolves over time, regardless of its starting place. Living systems move constantly through changes, often repeated patterns of change (stable attractors are a kind of "rut" in non-technical language), even though they may not pass through an identical path at each iteration.

In a sense, health is a particular behavioral pattern of motion (an attractor) that represents optimal complexity of the system in its environment. Disease is a different attractor pattern, in the context of the larger environment in which the individual lives. **At the level of scale of the person, healing is the ability to become unstuck from dysfunctional patterns (sickness=maladaptive recurrent patterns=ruts) and to shift persistently into more functional patterns of being (health=adaptable recurrent patterns).**

The graphical examples of different attractor patterns below might correspond to emergent disease (far left) versus wellness (far right) patterns for a particular network system. The examples shown in the figures are graphs modeling the social dynamics of business teams with track records, respectively, of poor, intermediate, and excellent productivity by objective standards. The dynamics traced are the patterns of interpersonal behaviors between group members as interconnected parts of the whole system, during a collaborative effort to develop a business plan.

Behaviors in the world are the expression of the system's relative level of functionality – of disease versus health. Some researchers are beginning to apply these same ideas at the level of an individual person to define human flourishing (wellness) or languishing (pre-illness and illness). It is important to note that "behavior" is both consciously and unconsciously expressed by the system as a whole.

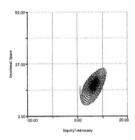
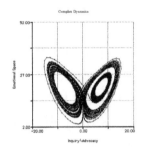
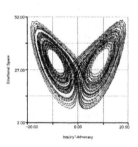

Figure 2-5A	Figure 2-5B	Figure 2-5C

Figure 2-5A
Graph of poor team dynamics of group with low productivity. Note the small, inflexible, restricted range of behavioral function within which the whole team gets stuck (point attractor pattern)

Figure 2-5B
Graph of mixed team dynamics of group with medium productivity. Note the variation between a wide range and a moderate range of function within which the whole team shows its behaviors (limit cycle to chaotic attractor pattern)

Figure 2-5C
Graph of good team dynamics of group with high productivity. Note the broader, more flexible and resilient variability of range in behavioral function within which the whole team can move in their interactions (Lorenz chaotic "butterfly" attractor pattern)

"The only difference between a rut and a grave is their dimensions."
~Ellen Glasgow

On the worse side of change — disease translates into a loss of optimal complexity in the complex living system dynamics as a whole – *i.e.*, excessive order (at the extreme, death itself) or excessive chaos in a complex system. With excessive order, the dynamical pattern of the system is not flexible enough to deal with environmental stressors or change as it arises. In a healthier system, there is dynamical flexibility to accommodate stressors and change.

"I don't believe one grows older. I think that what happens early on in life is that at a certain age one stands still and stagnates."
~T.S. Eliot

Chronic disease is a manifestation of being stuck in a pattern of being that is bad for you, *i.e.*, a dynamical rut. The pattern shows up in your biological, psychological, social, and spiritual ways of being, the successes and failures you manifest, the diseases and health you manifest. These ways of being are interwoven and interconnected. Whatever organ or organs are dysfunctional or damaged are not the basic problem. Symptoms are a sign of a larger problem.

You — that is, you as a whole system — are sick in your overall dynamical patterning, i.e., how you spontaneously function in your world. It is not a simple result of your conscious behaviors or mental state or a chemical change in your brain or a loss of heart muscle or a growth in your liver, lung or ovary. The body parts are just giving you Biofeedback with a capital B. At the same time, the lesson is that your chronic illness is not your fault, but it is the manifestation of the sum of your life, your choices, your genes, your ancestors' choices, and your environment.

> *"If you would attain to what you are not yet, you must always be displeased by what you are. For where you are pleased with yourself there you have remained. Keep adding, keep walking, keep advancing."*
> ~Saint Augustine

This is important to emphasize: **Blame is pointless. Change is the point.** Meaningful change as a whole being is your challenge. Finding the best ways for you to begin, maintain, and support change in your Self will lead to healing and better health in your parts. The goal is to find a way to free yourself from your disease ruts at your highest level of organization, that is, to **become the best you that you can be.**

If this book speaks some truths to you, then please read on and use the words as a guide. But know that you are and must be the steward of your own healing. You will need coaches, practitioners, doctors, healers, or teachers to nudge you along the way. You will want friends and family along for support. In the end, however, this healing process is, and can only be, your story. **You have to be you, to be healthy.**

"Whatever you are, be a good one."
~Abraham Lincoln

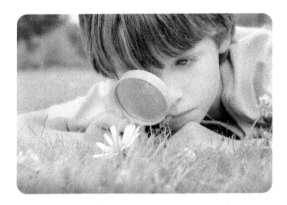

Figure 2-6

Chapter 2 Summary of Key Points

● A whole person is an indivisible, interconnected complex living network system, not a collection of separate body parts.

● Disease is a global problem in the person-system as a network, not a local symptom or problem in a body part. The local manifestation, *i.e.*, symptom, is a holographic picture of the global dysfunction in the person as a whole system.

● Change at any level of a network system leads to change at levels of organization above and below the initially affected level.

● As a complex living network system, a person is nonlinear (output is disproportionate to input) and dynamical (changing over time). Small interventions at hubs of the network can stimulate far-reaching changes throughout the rest of the network, for better or worse.

● Healing is getting unstuck and moving on to better patterns of being. In whole person healing, you as a nonlinear dynamical system are breaking free of stuckness, of repeated dysfunctional patterns of being (ruts) and shifting into lasting healthy patterns of being.

● In short, to be healthy, you have to become the best Self that you can be.

● You have to get unstuck, and you have to be You.

Chapter 3

Stuck in the Forest? Take Stock of your Illness and your Healing Dynamics

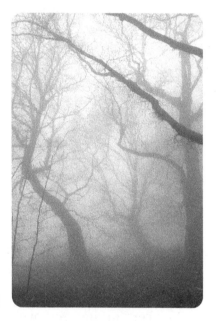

Figure 3-1

"Everyone who is born holds dual citizenship, in the kingdom of the well and in the kingdom of the sick. Although we all prefer to use only the good passport, sooner or later each of us is obliged, at least for a spell, to identify ourselves as citizens of that other place."
~Susan Sontag, *Illness as Metaphor*

If you are now thinking that this is just another book that tells you to pull your act together and get yourself well, you are wrong. **You cannot will disease to stop or go away by brute force.** If you are now thinking that I am going to propose some "amazing new treatment" for everyone with a particular disease, you are wrong. Rather, disease is a much more difficult challenge than most of us can overcome by willpower or taking a specific magic pill or visiting a powerful healer.

Disease is part of life, part of the lessons we are each here to learn about freedom, about not putting ourselves into this or that box.

"The obstacle is the path."
~Zen Proverb

Just as you are a unique individual in the universe, **what you will need to heal is most likely unique to you.** It will be some package of treatments, events, and people at a certain time and over time that will be the answer for you. And for that package to help you undergo the most lasting and complete healing, you will most likely need to make changes in how you live your life. Not superficial changes, not new diets or exercise programs. Real changes in your being.

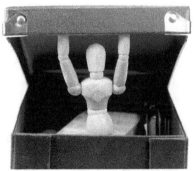

Figure 3-2

To do so, you will have to leave your comfort zone of the familiar and the comfortable ways of being in some profound way. Outer changes might occur in your relationships, your job, your lifestyle, your habits, your living and working environment. But the inner changes will underlie the outer ones, and the inner movement will shift you in how you are in your world.

You are expressing disease because you, as a dynamical system, are dysfunctional within the larger system/ environment in which you live. Given your personal social, physical, and/or chemical environmental context, you are not being the best You that you can be.

If you can change the context – move to a new city or change jobs or get a divorce from a bad marriage, you might recover. But, **if you can change yourself, you will recover. Sometimes the context will change as a part of the inner changes, sometimes not. What changes is how to relate to the world around you.**

> *"Vitality shows in not only the ability to persist but the ability to start over."*
> ~F. Scott Fitzgerald

Movie Metaphor Moment

In the movie *Groundhog Day*, Bill Murray's character Phil Connors is a callous, selfish, and insensitive TV news reporter who is consumed with himself. He finds himself stuck in an endless daily repetition of the same wintery day's experiences, *i.e.*, Groundhog Day, in Punxsutawney, Pennsylvania. This city touts itself as "The Original Weather Capitol of the World Since 1887," where the groundhog Punxsutawney Phil may or may not see his shadow that day — and thus predict the beginning of Spring. Phil Connors finally starts changing as he goes through the same day's events over and over. He begins to behave differently in encounters with people as he starts to recognize and meet other people's needs and respond to their feelings instead of his own selfish interests. Finally, once he has been sufficiently transformed by his experiences, he wakes up on the day after Groundhog Day. He is fully his best self, an unstuck man, ready to return to reality and experience the next days after Groundhog Day with his fresh perspective. Our diseases are also ruts, and we repeat the pattern until we find a way to shift the experience and become our best selves. Certain treatments are more likely to help you get unstuck and on your way.

You might have to change both your context and your-self. Can you make these kinds of changes by deciding to do them and just doing them? Maybe, though not many people can. More likely, some personalized package of care will help you make the changes and support you through them until they become an integral part of you.

To be sure, spontaneous healing does occur, as does healing from treatment with an isolated intervention, be it conventional or alternative. Miracles do occur, and some people get to stay the same and nonetheless give up their disease.

At the same time, in my practice I used to watch in amazement and sadness when dozens of patients with a chronic disease would flock to a particular treatment after word spread through their support network that one of their own had experienced a remarkable recovery from the "same" health problem during the treatment. I never saw the others respond as miraculously or as well to the same treatment as did the one person for whom it appeared to make such a difference. It was as though that one person was poised and ready to respond, that the treatment somehow spoke to his or her condition in some unique, well-matched way.

The other patients were apparently not poised to respond to that treatment, and its language was unfortu-nately foreign to their conditions. I believe that the person with the miracle recovery did need the treatment they received at the time to experience their excellent outcome. It wasn't a meaningless coincidence, but it may have been a meaningful synchronicity. The inner and outer circumstances were all set just right when the treatment arrived into his or her life. And the treatment arrived, because of the readiness of the person and the environmental context.

The point is that health care providers, healers, and treatments are external to you. Most of us need them to heal. However, they are a necessary but not sufficient element of the healing process. True healing must come from within, assisted and/or nurtured by the external help. At just the right moment.

I have also seen people undergo subtle energy treatments by extraordinarily talented healers who could somehow force the person's physical body to recover from disease instantly or overnight. And typically, I have heard that the same person enjoyed their newfound health for a few hours, days, weeks, or months – but then the condition returned. In my view, the problem returned because the person had not truly changed, and the disease was an expression of their internal dynamics, not some superimposed external misfortune that another person could remove for them.

The goal is to put together your personal treatment program in a way that will move you closer to inner readiness to heal and position you to have an extraordinary healing response to the package of care you assemble.

> *"Our repugnance to death increases in proportion to our consciousness of having lived in vain."*
> ~William Hazlitt, *On the Love of Life*

What's in Your Dynamics?

Table 3-1

The Disease Stuckness Quiz – What's in Your Dynamics?

Disease Stuckness Quiz

On a scale of 1 to 5, with 1 = not true for me, and 5 = very true for me, rate yourself for each item below. Add up your scores when you are done.

Question	Your Rating
1. I have had a chronic disease from early in life (before my mid-life years).	_____
2. My biological parents and grandparents were sick with serious diseases much of their lives.	_____
3. I am the kind of person who stays in an intimate relationship or a close friendship with someone even when it no longer nurtures me.	_____
4. I find myself in repetitive patterns in at least one area of my life that seem to end badly for me again and again.	_____

5. The kind of chronic disease(s) that I have developed affects my brain or nervous system, or another major organ. _____

6. I rarely catch colds or flu. _____

7. I must take at least one prescription drug regularly. _____

8. I feel that my life is in a rut. _____

9. It is hard for me to bounce back from setbacks or big changes in my life. _____

10. I have to stay in my current job for the money, the benefits, and/or the security. _____

11. I need to do certain things as much as I can or I do not feel well (*e.g.*, exercise, control my eating, swallow my anger – or vent my anger, get out – or stay home – more). _____

12. I should work harder – or, its opposite – I should take it easier. _____

TOTAL DISEASE STUCKNESS SCORE _____

The maximum score is 60. A score above 36 suggests significant amounts of stuckness. The higher your score, the more stuck you are likely to be in your chronic disease – and your life, of which the mental, emotional, or physical disease is one major manifestation. Feeling a need or having to do –

or not do – something most of the time limits your freedom. A lower disease stuckness score suggests that the right individualized treatments will move you along more readily and perhaps faster than someone with a higher score.

Do not despair, however – you can usually get unstuck no matter how high your score, unless you are in your final moments of this life. A higher score simply means that it may take more time and persistence from you to get free and stay free of your disease rut. And even when cure is not possible, people can and do heal, especially in their final moments of life.

Use your Disease Stuckness Quiz score as a general guide: (a) to help you set up the extent of your treatment program. The higher your score, the more likely it is that you will need a full program at multiple levels of the system to get yourself unstuck and sustain you in making lasting changes to heal. With a lower score, a simpler program with one modality may be sufficient; (b) to prepare you for how long it might take to see significant change.

The higher your score, the more likely it is that you will want to give each treatment option and yourself a longer period of time to heal, *e.g.*, perhaps on the order of a year or more. With a lower score, the simpler program may produce good results in only a few months.

Some complementary medicine practitioners describe health as freedom at every level of being – spiritual, social, mental, emotional, physical. A truly healthy person may catch a cold or feel down for a short time under stress, but he or she recovers quickly. If a life situation generates problems, a healthy person finds a way to reframe, change, or move out of or past the situation. Taking an occasional aspirin for a headache is not the issue here; rather, having to take a drug every day to stay alive represents an extreme loss of freedom at a physical plane. The freedom expresses itself as resilience.

This is not to say that you should stop your medications and pretend that you are fine. Denying illness or making believe you are healthy is not the same thing as being healthy. For example, many diabetics try to ignore their dietary requirements and let their blood sugar soar out of control. They pay a dear price in the form of suffering, complications, disability, and early death for their denial. Rather, disease and its necessary treatment mean that you have a significant amount of physical stuckness that you cannot – and should not – try to pretend away. Being sick, but denying that you are sick, is itself a life box within which you can trap yourself.

"Here I am trying to live, or rather, I am trying to teach the death within me how to live."
~Jean Cocteau

For most people, chronic disease itself puts them into a box – as much for the symptoms as for the treatments. When you are diagnosed with a chronic disease, confronting your physical limitations, disability, and death itself is often frightening and unsettling. That point in time is also a potential tipping point for you in your life – you are un-settled, un-stuck in a sense, and the situation offers an opportunity to make changes. Sometimes you are too sick for a while to do much other than survive the best you can.

However, as with all of life's big challenges, the person who faces the fear and uncertainty and carries on, determined to survive for some larger purpose, with a sense of meaning and goals, is more likely to pull through the disease experience and move on into a new, often healthier, way of life than someone who gives up. What is encouraging is that certain types of health care options may be more likely to help you take advantage of the unstuckness, *i.e.*, survive, make changes – many gradual and even imperceptible until you look back at them, maintain the beneficial changes, and even thrive in a hard-won new freedom of being. Your goal is to change your everyday patterns, not just a few fleeting moments.

"Things do not change, we change."
~Henry David Thoreau

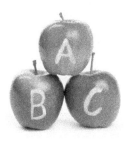

Chapter 3 Summary of Key Points

- Disease is a manifestation of being stuck in a rut – that is, in a recurring dynamical pattern that is less than optimal for you as an individual network system in the context of your larger environment.

- Your response to a chronic disease diagnosis may in itself trigger a window of unstuckness – or not – as you adjust to facing impairments, disability, and ultimately mortality.

- When you become unstuck, (a) you may go on to make changes in yourself and your circumstances, move past disease patterns into healthier patterns, and even transform at a spiritual level or (b) you may relapse into old familiar patterns that are again stuck in chronic disease.

- Using your health care options from a whole systems orientation to support you into and through unstuckness into full healing and transformation will favor healing and transformation rather than relapse.

- Healing can occur suddenly or gradually. You may be less aware of the process when it is gradual, but you will be able to look back when you emerge from the fog of transition and see that you live in new, healthier patterns.

- Health is freedom at the spiritual, mental, emotional, and physical levels of being.

Chapter 4

ASSESS — You CAN Get There from Here: Discover All of Your Options

Figure 4-1

"The Scarecrow crosses his arms and points in both directions – SCARECROW: "...go both ways!"
~From *The Wizard of Oz* Screenplay

Have you ever seen the cure of the week for XYZ disease? Next week someone else will proclaim that they are Professor Marvel or the Wizard of Oz and have The Answer to your condition (different from last week's cure). Worse than that, have you ever found that one practitioner tells you do one thing and another provider tells you to do the opposite for the same condition – or tells you that the first thing is just bad for you. How do you judge? It is very difficult. This chapter offers you a way to think about your health care options as you make decisions.

> "When you come to a fork in the road, take it."
> ~Yogi Berra

World Views of Nature and Health Care Options

The Conventional Medical View. Mainstream conventional or Western medicine is the politically dominant form of health care in developed nations. The central world view assumption about nature in Western medicine is that the person is a physical entity in which some external cause produces an effect (disease manifestations). Conventional treatment consists of doing something at the local physical level to block the cause from acting on the body. Disease is considered a foreign enemy attacking the body in a particular place. Conventional physicians rely on pharmaceutical drugs as their main tool. The focus of conventional medicine is looking for a single cause to produce a single effect.

However, it also is possible to use nutritional supplements and herbs or botanical supplements as though they were drugs. Many health care providers and patients can hang onto their world view that nature is just a physical place in which disease is an external enemy – and they simply substitute natural products for drugs.

The natural products may — or may not — be safer than the drugs, as supplements are also much less regulated and standardized. It is less certain what you are actually taking. With thoughtful research, however, you can find safe and effective supplements. How you use them is another matter.

At the interface between Western medicine and much of complementary and alternative medicine (CAM) is preventive medicine, with a foundational or bridging role in promoting health through exercise, good diet, regular sleep, and positive habits (keeping close to your ideal weight, using a seat belt in a car, not smoking, or using recreational drugs, drinking in moderation). These are important basics in all health care to foster optimum healing and maintain good health.

At the cutting edge of conventional medicine, genetics researchers recognize that individual differences in genetic potential increase or decrease the risk for developing a disease in the first place. In some ways, Western medicine is moving slowly toward a greater preventive approach, that is, shutting off the "bad" genes that make you individually vulnerable to certain external diseases (the problems that environmental factors could activate in you).

One current concern about the genetics approach is that doctors are planning to micromanage specific genes. Many doctors are still not thinking very much about the larger implications of turning one gene on and another gene off for the person as a whole system. Researchers have begun to realize that most chronic diseases are multifactorial, even at the genetic level. Their first successes are most likely to come from genetic diseases with a single or simple genetic "mistake" underlying them.

However, the most common chronic diseases appear to be far more complex than a single genetic flaw. Chronic diseases involve multiple genes, probably even different ones in different people, and many interacting factors from the environment play a role. The rest of the person as a nonlinear dynamical network system might or might not end up out of balance with other downstream complications of gene therapy that tries to alter a specific local problem.

The Western conventional medical way is to do things to the body parts to make them work "better." Most of us with chronic diseases need to take Western drugs to get by in everyday life. Western conventional medicine can be life-saving and invaluable with trauma and many acute illnesses, as well as in replacing irreparably damaged body parts or lost body fluids or blocking unbearable pain and lessening discomfort from various symptoms.

However, Western conventional care is not geared to curing or healing chronic disease. Rather, conventional care is set up to control symptoms of chronic disease, that is, the local manifestations. It is far better suited to treating acute diseases such as infections, in which a germ (bacteria, virus, etc.) that is not part of the person per se has taken hold in the physical body which has become susceptible to the specific germ. Western care is focused on treating from the outside in.

"The art of medicine consists in amusing the patient while nature cures the disease."
~Voltaire

However, many CAM healing systems see chronic disease as a deeper problem with multiple causes that all possible "right living" may not prevent. A host of interactive factors may still enable the expression of disease. Inherited disease vulnerabilities (*e.g.*, through genetics), unintentional dietary errors, environmental toxins, negative social settings with perceived daily hassles and stressful major life events (negative traumas or even major positive changes) can foster development of disease.

The spiritual challenges that you face in life and any impaired resilience in throwing off their effects to bounce back may play out in the specifics of these factors and lead to development of disease.

The CAM Whole-System-Oriented View. Many CAM therapies, even ones that are not derived from the Eastern cultures, have a different way of conceptualizing the world of nature and of healing. These therapies intervene to allow the network system to heal itself from within and thereby work better overall. **Whole systems-oriented care is focused on healing the person from the inside out.** The complexity of living systems makes it hard or impossible to find a simple single cause for events in the system.

Table 4-1 shows you the levels into which health care options fall. Each has its own implicit assumptions, world view philosophies, and science behind it. Unfortunately, it is possible to use many of the CAM health care options in a conventional local way, that is, to force the body parts to stop manifesting disease.

For example, one Western way to use guided imagery tells one cell to attack and kill another cell within the person. A more systems-based way to use guided imagery or various forms of art expression asks the body part to dialogue with the whole person, tell the person what the larger message of the symptom or the disease is, and advise the best way to resolve the imbalance or problem for highest good of the person as a whole.

People who have used biofeedback can tell you that trying to make a body part behave in a certain way does not work. Trying to make something happen rather than let something happen causes stress in your mind and your body, and you cannot achieve the goal.

You have to allow the biofeedback from the body part teach you when you are passing through the desired state of being – then the equipment lets you know whenever you have achieved it. You can allow, but not force, the desired state to occur more often and more reliably.

It is also possible to use mind-body techniques, subtle energy therapies, or even prayer in a specific Western-based way of attacking the disease. That is, to use the mind or external energy or ask the Higher Power to force the body to stop manifesting the disease. Such treatments are usually either temporary in benefit or damaging to the rest of the whole person (the network system). The risk of harm to the extended network of the person is something that many individuals — some providers and many patients — do not realize as they take their Western conventional medical world view into the CAM arena.

Interestingly, on the one hand, some research on prayer even suggests that the more effective way to pray is non-directedly and globally for the universal network system – *i.e.*, to ask for "Thy Will be done," rather than directedly, to specify a local desired outcome. On the other hand, many experienced herbalists would object to being placed in the same category with drugs and will say that they use botanical agents to treat the whole person and restore balance within the overall system, not to drug a symptom into oblivion.

The point is that most CAM therapies can be used in either way – one that applies the Western conventional world view that disease comes from outside, arises locally, and can be attacked – or a whole systems world view that disease arises from within the overall person, as a message from the Self to the Self that the whole system is out of balance and needs deep and profound change first at the deepest levels of your being.

It is important to emphasize that the table is an oversimplification. The world of health care options does not fall neatly into a set of boxes any more than people do. Practitioners of various types of health care options will probably question the placement of their particular form of intervention in a particular category.

In reality, every health care intervention will have effects on every other level of the person as a network system, above and below the organizational level of the person (see Chapter 2). The categories are only a rough guide as to how to understand the potential role of a given level of health care options for your chronic disease.

The Resources chapter at the end of this book provides brief definitions of leading types of health care options and where to find more information about options listed in Table 4-1. **As you review the table, note that you are zooming out in your world view perspective from the micro-physical/chemical plane to the universal plane of reality as you consider the different health care options running down the first column. Think big picture, then fill in the details.**

Table 4-1.

Levels of Health Care

LEVEL OF HEALTH CARE OPTIONS	TYPES	WORLD VIEW ASSUMPTIONS
Biochemical/ Biological	Drugs, nutrients, botanicals (herbs)	External physical causes lead to physical effects in the local body parts – thereby causing disease or treating disease.
Preventive Foundations	Exercise, diet, sleep	Strengthening the person physically reduces the risk of developing disease.
Structural, manual manipulation	Osteopathy, chiropractic, massage	The physical body is an indivisible, interactive system. Putting the physical structure in proper alignment permits healing from within.
Mind-body	Meditation, yoga, biofeedback, guided imagery, journaling	Non-physical mind and physical body are inter-active parts of a person as a whole network system. It is possible to tap inner wisdom to foster healing.

Subtle Energy	Therapeutic Touch, Healing Touch, Reiki, Johrei, Qi Gong	People are interactive parts of a larger non-physical reality in which subtle energy can be channeled through one person (healer) to another (patient). It is possible to "send" external energy to a person to foster inner healing or to force disease from the outside to stop manifesting.
Constitutional	Homeopathy, Traditional Chinese Medicine/Acupuncture, Ayurveda	People are unique indivisible network systems within larger network systems comprised of both physical and non-physical parts in interaction. Disease begins at the individual spiritual level and expresses itself dynamically through the energetic and physical levels of the person. Healing occurs from within outward and involves the person network-system as a whole at every level of organization.

Spiritual	Intention or prayer	People are unique inter-active parts of the larger complex universal spiritual whole or non-local cosmic consciousness, an Infinite One. We each have our role and our place in the universe. Disease and healing are local properties of people as natural parts of the Infinite.

This perspective gives you a big picture view of chronic disease and health care options. Some people may wish to look at the process from top down; others from bottom up in a hierarchy. The likelihood is that there is a circle joining bottom to top rather than a straight line going in one direction or the other – and thus, you can end up in the same place whether you begin at the top or the bottom. What is likely, however, is that you will have to choose the providers and therapies that make up your treatment program. And your healing will involve much more than going to providers and undergoing treatments.

You may or may not be ready to look at the whole big picture as this book presents it or to question your own assumptions about health and disease. If you are ready, then

move on to Chapter 5. Your next step is to select and imple-
ment your individual plan for healing from chronic disease.

---

*"The illiterate of the 21st century will not be
those who cannot read and write, but those who
cannot learn, unlearn, and relearn."*
~Alvin Toffler

Chapter 4 Summary of Key Points

- The Western conventional medical world-oriented view is that disease comes from outside and attacks the body parts. Treatments must consider the situation as a war, with good guys on the inside (the patient) fighting bad guys on the outside (the disease, the symptoms).

- An alternative whole systems world view is that disease comes from within. The disease is just an expression of the whole Self that reveals inner disharmonies that must be rebalanced gently and in accord with the individualized essence of the person who has the disease.

- Most health care options can be used in a Western conventional medical way to attack disease as something from outside the body, even though they are called "CAM."

- The larger set of health care options other than conventional drugs can be used in either a conventional local or systems-oriented way. It is the choice of the consumer, the patient, how to proceed.

Chapter 5

BALANCE — There's No Place Like
Home: Set your Healing Intention

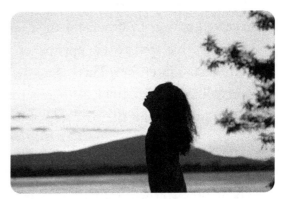

Figure 5-1

"A man is what he thinks about all day long."
~Ralph Waldo Emerson

The dictionary defines intention in general as "a course of action that one intends to follow," "an aim or objective." Ironically, in conventional medicine, the word intention means "the process by which a wound heals." In a much broader sense, for healing from chronic disease, setting the intention to heal is the overarching first step in creating your program and putting the healing process into motion.

In setting this type of intention, you are asking the universe, cosmic consciousness, or God – however you are most comfortable addressing the "highest" level of infinite reality – to help you achieve the goal of healing.

A recent survey of CAM use in the U.S. found that prayer for health was the most widely-used form of "CAM" in the previous year (43% prayed for their own health; 24% received prayers by others for their own health). You can consider this step to be praying or you can consider it setting your intention. This is a matter of labels with which you feel most comfortable. Whatever the label, setting your intention to heal is the core step of the overall plan.

It is up to the universe to figure out the details. You identify the goal, that is, healing. You may have some ideas about how you will start to go about operationalizing the steps along the way, and you will need to take those steps. When the intention is clear, the process will take over and lead you into whatever experiences, treatments, and people will ultimately be involved in your healing.

Make no assumptions that what or whomever is right for you now will remain right for you throughout the process. Remember, you are a dynamical being, ever-changing, expressing your free will in the context of a larger, a much larger environment.

There is no one right way to set an intention. It may be more common to do so in a quiet contemplative moment when you are fully present, without distractions of daily life. You may be alone or with someone you care about and who cares for you. For you, it may require a silent resolution, a statement out loud to yourself, a written diary entry, or a statement to a loved one. What is important is to aim as globally as you can in setting the intention, *i.e.*, that you are healing as a whole (not that just your body part is healing). As Larry Dossey, MD has said of prayer – *Be Careful What You Pray For, You Just Might Get It.* In this case, your goal is systemic healing, not just conventional medical local healing.

In other words, play big, not small. If you ask for small changes in body parts, you just might get those. If you ask for whole person healing as part of the Universe's big picture, you just might get a transformation.

Setting an intention reflects clarity, simplicity, focus, largeness, love, determination, and positiveness. Bring together your feelings and your resolve in the moment of commitment to the intention.

Your intention is speaking to your deepest subconscious and unconscious mind and the larger non-local universal consciousness. Phrase the intention in a positive manner – that is, "I am healing, I am whole at the physical, mental, emotional, and spiritual levels of my being, for the highest and best good of all" (rather than saying, "I don't have disease XYZ any more"). Aim for the most transcendent level with your intention.

Some people find it helpful to reinforce intentions with affirmations that they repeat to themselves regularly, for example, just before going to sleep at night or during free moments earlier in the day. Affirmations help reprogram your mind to support your intention. Affirmations may help you avoid becoming deflected away from your intention when your environment sends everyday challenges to you.

If you want to use a particular script for setting an intention, you might look at one of several books and resources mentioned at the end of this book, including Wayne Dyer's *The Power of Intention* or Joe Vitale's *The Attractor Factor*. You can also get an e-workbook on affirmations at www.BestAffirmations.com. Scripts can be very helpful if you feel uncertain how to phrase your intention. However, the words must feel genuine for you – if your spiritual or religious beliefs, your world view, or other considerations make you uncomfortable with specific wording for an intention or affirmation, do not use it. Create your own. This is your unique moment to be honest and clear with yourself in your own context.

*"If the highest aim of a captain were to preserve
his ship, he would keep it in port forever."*
~Saint Thomas Aquinas

Finally, after zooming out to the most global level to set
your intention, then consider the next levels of network
system organization on down. You cannot heal selfishly.
**You can only heal unselfishly into your full role within
the universe.** When you set your healing intention, intend
that your healing will free you to fulfill your life's purpose,
to give to others in whatever way you are uniquely here to
give. This does not mean that you must become a Mother
Teresa or Gandhi or leader of nations. **It means that you
find clarity about your niche in the universe and be your
best self in your niche.**

"Live your beliefs and you can turn the world around."
~Henry David Thoreau

Chapter 5 Summary of Key Points

- Start your healing program at the highest level of organization, that is, with the intention to heal globally (rather than in a specific body part). Play big, not small.

- Phrase your intention with clarity, simplicity, focus, largeness, love, and positive feeling.

- Support your intention by repeating affirmations daily.

- Let the process take over and be open to how the universe will work out the details with you and for you.

Chapter 6

COORDINATE — Design Your Own Yellow
Brick Road and Get Moving

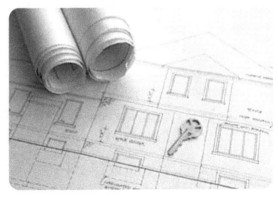

Figure 6-1

*"Things alter for the worse spontaneously, if they
be not altered for the better designedly."*
~Francis Bacon

Organizing and Coordinating Your Treatment

In this chapter, you will get a general overview of how to choose and combine the health care options outlined in Chapter 4. As you will see, using your health care options in a systems-oriented way (Chapter 2) can provide you with your own Yellow Brick Road. This is no time for stuckness in making new health care decisions. Now is the time for getting yourself unstuck and supporting your Self through the healing process (Chapter 3).

The basic principle is to address your chronic disease through multiple coordinated levels of intervention that together keep your whole system changing toward better health at multiple levels.

Trying combinations of treatments that mostly fall into the same level of options is less likely to produce optimal results. For example, adding more and more nutritional or botanical supplements (Biochemical level of options) but no other type of treatment from the other levels of options is only likely to become expensive without getting you unstuck and moving along toward systemic health.

An exception might be if your disease is due to nutritional deficiencies, and supplements are all you need to correct the deficiencies.

However, for the typically complex chronic diseases of modern life such as inflammatory conditions, autoimmunity, heart and blood vessel problems, cancer, arthritis, and multi-system conditions such as chronic fatigue syndrome or fibromyalgia, a multi-system treatment program package is usually preferable to an overly narrow one that speaks to only one level of your overall system.

Coordinating Your Systems-Oriented Treatment Planning

First, the prioritizing of interventions is the reverse order of the list in Chapter 4. That is, you will start with the spiritual level of prayer and/or intention, which is singular and focused. Your intention to heal sets in motion the new pattern of change that you will undertake. It provides the umbrella for the package of care. Then you select from the different levels of options below the spiritual to fill in the ways in which you will work to get yourself unstuck and moving in a healing direction as a whole system.

Constitutional Systemic and Subtle Energy Treatment Options. Here you will select whichever one form of constitutional treatment (Chinese medicine/acupuncture or classical homeopathy or Ayurveda) appeals most to you, is accessible to you in terms of provider availability and costs, and has the best evidence of helping in your specific condition (see the Resources section at the end for brief definitions and links to additional books and information for disease-specific guidance).

Constitutional systems of care tend to have long historical roots for hundreds to thousands of years. Chinese medicine, which includes acupuncture, is from China, classical homeopathy from Germany (Europe), and Ayurveda from India. **All of these systems describe the person as an intact whole, an interconnected network, in which the goal of treatment is to restore balance of function between the body parts throughout the whole system and harmony with the larger environment around the person (the natural, social, and transcendent worlds). Using a constitutional treatment that addresses the core illness process within you as a whole is the most powerful way to stimulate deep healing throughout your being.**

It is best not to start more than one constitutional option of treatment at a time, as these are the most powerful forms of systemic treatment for chronic disease. Each constitutional program has its own transitional processes in stimulating healing that proceed best without disruption by another such process, especially in the beginning.

Can you combine two or more types of constitutional care? The answer is a cautious yes, though the combination requires collaboration between your providers and added skills and awareness of how you respond to each treatment. As time passes, the beneficial changes from systemic treatment become ingrained in your dynamics and patterns, making it easier to put you back on course if something happens to set you back or off track again.

Be aware that providers differ widely not only in their skill and experience, but also in how they use these treatment options. **Ask if the way in which the treatment** option is given is constitutional, that is, treating you as a whole indivisible system, rather than controlling local symptoms (the more Western conventional medical mind-set way of treating disease).

A clue in that area is whether or not the practitioner can give you a unified diagnosis and a coordinated treatment plan within their system of care for your entire pattern of problems rather than just one of them. You want to avoid practitioners who mainly use acupuncture or homeopathy or Ayurvedic methods to treat disease locally at a body part. You may need local treatment during acute health crises or flare-ups of your chronic illness, but your greatest progress stems from gradual constitutional treatment over time rather than treating one crisis after the next.

Similarly, subtle energy healing as an option is a complex topic. Many persons are capable of affecting a person's subtle energy body in major ways and can further develop their capabilities with relatively brief training programs. However, many such individuals are less well trained in understanding the systemic implications of their abilities, and many have no background in any form of health care (a common exception is nurses who do therapeutic touch or healing touch).

Some energy healers send well-intentioned general positive energy to you overall that can help you superficially for a while, but likely cannot heal a deep-seated chronic disease. Some are very powerful in their ability and can force the physical manifestations of a specific disease to go away by blocking the energetic patterns that underlie the expression in the physical body — But they are not aware of the risks of suppressing the disease manifestations into the rest of the person as an indivisible network.

For example, I once heard an energy healer describe a client whose long-standing pain and disability from a leg injury had stopped in a matter of days, under subtle energy healing focused on recovery of the leg. At first I congratulated the healer and asked how the client was doing now, a year later. What she said distressed me – she acknowledged that the client's leg was still pain-free with much better functionality, but now the client was suffering from horrible panic attacks, unable to leave home.

So, the treatment was powerful and seemingly "effective" – but it was directed to healing a body part (the leg), not the person as a whole. As a result, the deepest disturbance was simply blocked from expressing itself in the leg – encouraging it to move deeper into the person, up to the level of the brain. Then the disturbance in the person as a whole system had taken on the form of panic disorder and agoraphobia. This was not really a desirable outcome – but neither the healer nor the client realized the possible connection. A different healer who incorporated an understanding of the need to heal the leg in the context of the person as a whole might have produced a very different result — healing both the underlying disturbance and the leg as a manifestation.

Distant parts of the network (the rest of the body) may experience adverse outcomes as a result of the suppression of local symptoms in one part.

At the same time, some energy healers have a true gift for helping people at a profoundly spiritual and integrated level. The treatment they provide is potentially as valuable in your overall package of care as any of the constitutional systems of treatment.

As a result, it is always important to do your homework about any provider to whom you entrust your health and well-being, but especially a subtle energy practitioner. If you prefer this approach instead of the formal constitution-ally-oriented systems of treatment, by all means do so, but with the above caveats in mind. Ask questions – re-assess how you are doing as treatment proceeds. It is your life and your body to heal.

Mind-Body Treatment Options. You can support these first two components of your care by adding whatever form(s) of mind-body approaches appeal to you (*e.g.*, journaling, affirmations, guided imagery, hypnosis, biofeedback). **These approaches are often very helpful to support your healing intention by reprogramming your subconscious mind,** especially for people who find it easy to generate imagery and/or who are verbal, depending on the method chosen.

Some research suggests that there are individual differences in personality types in terms of who benefits from specific types of mind-body interventions. For example, absorption is a genetically-determined trait involving openness to new experiences, high intrinsic spirituality, high hypnotizability, and the capacity to lose oneself in an inner or outer experience (*e.g.*, a sunset or a book or movie).

In people with chronic vascular headaches such as migraine, those who scored high on a questionnaire for absorption responded better to guided imagery than to biofeedback. In contrast, their peers who scored low on the same absorption scale responded better to biofeedback than to the imagery.

These observations suggest that we may someday be able to steer people with more certainty to the specific types of a treatment option that have the best chance of helping them as individuals. Genes determine personality traits, which means that personality reflects real biological differences in the brain and body from one person to another. For now, it appears likely that people with high or low trait absorption may need different types of treatments to maximize their recovery from chronic disease.

Structural/Manual Manipulation Treatment Level of Options. Especially if you have any musculoskeletal problems, the manual manipulation methods make great sense as well at this point. Whole systems of care such as osteopathy have a philosophical approach to the person that inherently views the body as comprised of interconnected, interrelated pathways. **Getting the physical body into alignment by a manual manipulation method of treatment is permissive**

for healing throughout the system overall. Subtle energy flows better; physical discomforts resolve.

Constitutional and energetic treatments are particularly complementary with manual manipulation treatments and vice versa – that is, positioning the physical body pathways properly enables constitutional/energy treatments to move past physical blocks and exert their best effects, whereas constitutional/energy treatments can help the physical body hold the healthier positioning of soft tissue and bones from manual manipulation treatments longer.

***Preventive and Biochemical Levels of Options.* Finally, make sure that you are doing at least the fundamentals of supporting your physical body through the preventive level of options — regular exercise, health-promoting diet, and nutritional supplements as appropriate to your age and condition.** A good multivitamin/mineral supplement, for example, is a basic for most people. Evidence suggests that such supplements are especially important for people with various chronic diseases to reduce their susceptibility to acute infections and to later life complications.

Your intention from Chapter 5 is firm, clear, unwavering. Paradoxically, even as you leave the details up to the universe, you still need to set some of the details in motion for Chapter 6 (that is, you will be selecting the elements of your individualized package of care). You can and must do things to help yourself.

As the adage goes, "God helps those who help themselves." You can only start, of course. **The details of the process are subject to revision – frequent or infrequent — as you go, based on the feedback you receive from your world and your experiences as you move along the path.** Practitioners and/or treatments may or may not be helpful, but doing nothing and just expecting a miracle is unlikely to yield favorable results.

Your involvement in designing your plan may mean that you will move on from one provider to a different one within the same treatment option, from one treatment option to a different one within a level (*e.g.*, from guided imagery to biofeedback), or just from one version of a treatment option to a different one (*e.g.*, one style of acupuncture to another). **Healing is a growth process.** Treatments, forms of treatments, and providers may be right for you at one point in the process but not in another.

The What, The How, The Who of Health Care Options

Health care options include a what (name or class of therapy), a how (particular school or style of the therapy), and a who (particular provider). All health care occurs in a context — the larger context of your life. Although you may see your health as separate from your life context, it is not. Health and disease are very much interwoven into the fabric of your life.

That is why you hear about people who undergo miraculous cures of their diseases talking about changes in themselves that go far beyond the resolution of a health problem. Your health care is simply a local focus for you to get the help to get out on your Yellow Brick Road to healing.

The Who of Your Healing Program. Your program will most likely involve you and professional providers in selecting and implementing various tools for healing. The Who is variable. You will always be the person making the decisions as to whom to involve in your care. Some of the way, however, you may also learn about a valuable self-care tool from a provider or a book or website or a friend or family member.

Some of the tools will involve self-care, not a professional provider. You may identify a form of a tool that is helpful for you to incorporate into your program. You do not necessarily need a provider for every aspect of your health care. In chronic disease, research shows that one of the most important aspects of improving your sense of self-efficacy and your outcome is learning how to manage day to day aspects of living well and coping with disease-related challenges for yourself. Expecting a professional to be there all the time is not only unrealistic, it misses the point of growing through facing challenges on your own.

To the extent that a health care option depends on a particular provider's judgment of what is wrong and what treatment is needed, things may go better or worse. In the ideal, each provider is equally qualified in terms of technical training and preparation to help you to the maximum possible and in personal qualities with which you resonate. In the real world, providers are people with their own technical and personal strengths and weaknesses.

In the real world, you may or may not develop a good relationship and communication channel with a particular provider. A provider may have what appear to be good tools technically, but difficult to work with in the therapeutic relationship. Another provider may be very caring and compassionate but still not have the perspective, knowledge, or tools that will help you the most.

If you happen to find both the relationship and the tools in the same provider, rejoice and partner with them in your healing process. However, some providers, even the most talented, may also be so bound up in ego issues about needing to help you and taking credit for your recovery that they have their own unresolved issues that are not yours to take on.

For your healing, seek selfless compassionate healers who have only your highest and best good as their intention, not another notch on their therapeutic gun. Flee from providers who tell you that you must forsake all other care for them and their approach, as they have the only right and true answer for you. In some way, they are more of a cult leader than a true healer.

For an optimal healing environment, you will want your healers to relate to you in a way that makes you feel heard and understood. Although you may find that the turning point for your healing occurs under care with a particular person, you may also find that you need several different providers with different tools at the same time or over time.

Ideally, you will have a primary health care provider who understands how to integrate your treatment package. Some MDs and DOs (many of whom function essentially as conventional physicians and do not offer manual manipulative treatments) have such training in the sense that they have a strong background in Western conventional medicine, an important consideration. The limitation with them is often that they remain steeped in the conventional medical local mindset in their recommendations.

NDs (naturopaths) have a broad background in CAM modalities and a four-year naturopathic medical school training that emphasizes a world view of healing compatible with the systems orientation. Even so, NDs vary in the extent to which they use nutritional supplements and herbs in a systems-oriented versus conventional local manner. Ask about their approach.

Again, the situation is no one's fault if you need more than one person can provide, but it does require you to participate actively in the design and re-design of your program for getting whole and getting well. *It will be up to you to make informed choices of the what, the how, and the who in your health care, as well as the sequencing or timing of introducing each approach and each provider.*

The What and The How – Choosing the Tools of Your Healing Plan. It is also up to you to try out your treatment program and see if it helps you. **If a treatment option helps you, stay with it. If it does not lead to improvements in your health or it actually worsens your health, it is time to move on.** This sounds simple and obvious, but many people fall into a rut with this aspect of the process.

Many times, for example, I have seen people with a history of depression whose doctor had put them on a particular antidepressant drug. Even if they were still depressed a year or two later, no one – not the patient or any provider – had questioned whether or not it was time to move on to a different antidepressant drug or even to a different form of treatment. Somehow having connected the patient with a treatment that was supposed to help, even though it didn't, was mistakenly seen as enough by everyone involved. People settled for labels instead of results of treatment. This is the kind of situation where it is not enough to "get some help." It is up to you first, and your provider(s) second, to look objectively at whether or not the help is helping.

Most people with chronic disease are on conventional medical drugs when they start a fuller treatment plan. **Do not stop your prescription drugs before it is time to try to do so or in a manner that is counterproductive – and only make changes under the supervision of a qualified prescribing doctor.** Many people – but not all — find that they can gradually lower their medication doses or eventually stop the drugs altogether as other treatments begin to work.

However, it is not safe to reduce or stop your drugs too soon, at a time when nothing else has actually helped yet, unless the risk of doing so is minimal in your physician's judgment and you agree (*e.g.*, some increased pain or discomfort but not a flare in disease activity or death).

It is also often especially risky to stop drugs suddenly. Drugs are usually suppressing disease activity. Sudden removal of a drug from the body, which likely has generated a compensatory increase in disease activity behind the scenes to fight the drug effects, will unleash unopposed, increased disease activity. This is often dangerous and usually unnecessary.

Use common sense — I have heard of tragic cases of insulin-dependent diabetics, for instance, who stopped their insulin and died in diabetic coma with high blood sugars at the recommendation of an ignorant CAM provider who told them the new treatment would replace the insulin from the start and who misinterpreted the adverse effects of high blood sugar as a temporary healing crisis. It is easy enough to test your blood sugar and see if the insulin requirements go down – then it makes sense to reduce the drug accordingly in collaboration with the physician who prescribed it. If nothing changes, then you still need your insulin at the dose that your doctor originally prescribed.

For most chronic diseases, prioritize your choices. **The best way to get unstuck and to heal is to start with and prioritize the two most powerful levels of health care options. These are spiritual and constitutional.**

The other key practical decision is to continue your drugs for now, as discussed above. Continue the essential aspects of your biochemical level – *i.e.*, your Western conventional treatment, in consultation with your physician.

Table 6-1

Fill in your own personal, coordinated holistic healing care plan

LEVEL OF HEALTH CARE OPTIONS	Fill in Your Specific Choice (see Chapter 4)
1 Spiritual	Set one global healing intention:
2 Constitutional	Check or circle one: ❏ Acupuncture/Chinese medicine ❏ Classical homeopathy or ❏ Ayurveda
2a Subtle Energy	
3 Mind-Body	
4 Structural	

5 Preventive	
6 Biochemical/Biological	

Combining and Coordinating Options

Most people with chronic disease find that they must combine options down the vertical list. The number of interventions that makes sense usually runs from less to more as one goes from spiritual down to physical/biochemical.

That is, you will have only one overarching global intention to heal, but at the bottom of the list, you will likely be taking multiple medications for different body parts at first. You also will need multiple nutrients, not single nutrients. Nutrients work together in biochemical networks in the physical body and need each other in balanced amounts to optimize function.

Can or should you combine modalities at a given level? The answer is sometimes, but with increased caution about overdoing it and confusing your natural healing process. **More is not always better for non-drug therapies as much as for drug therapies, where undesirable drug-drug or drug-herb interactions are common.**

"To accomplish great things, we must not only act, but also dream, not only plan, but also believe."
~Anatole France

"Everything on the earth has a purpose, every disease an herb to cure it, and every person a mission."
~Mourning Dove [Christal Quintasket]

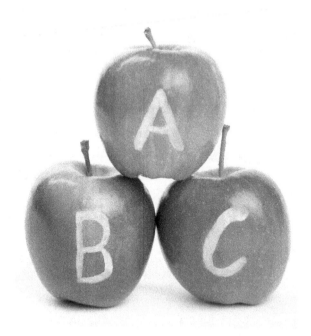

Chapter 6 Summary of Key Points

- Prioritize your levels of health care option to start with the spiritual (setting the healing intention) and then constitutional treatment to get unstuck.

- Fill in mind-body, structural, and finally biochemical levels of care for support in moving through unstuckness into lasting healthier change.

- Continue your conventional drugs until other treatments begin to improve your condition enough to work with your prescribing physician to gradually taper them. Do not stop your medications suddenly.

- Look at the What, the How, and the Who of your health care levels of options. Be prepared to try approaches or providers who may or may not be helpful – and to move on to the next option if they are not helping.

- If possible, find a primary provider MD/DO or ND who is a generalist and can work as a partner with you to make informed decisions as to the details of choosing your options and coordinating them.

  ○ Look for a generalist who understands the difference between a conventional medical and a systems mindset orientation to using health care options

Chapter 7

Pull Back the Curtain: Are You Better or Worse? Evaluate Your Progress

How Much Time To Give the Process

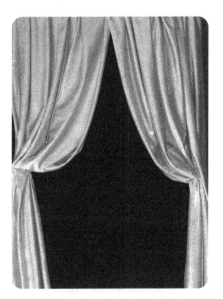

Figure 7-1

"Who ever is out of patience is out of possession of their soul."
~Francis Bacon

Overnight cures are wonderful miracles. They do happen. Rarely. **Gradual cures are far more common, especially with whole systems of CAM.** So, expect a possible miracle – or at least a solid improvement, but be prepared for a longer haul and perhaps less than a complete miracle. **Many people are healed but not cured. Aim for both cure and healing.** Do not settle for just coping better with your chronic disease unless you have given a systemic approach to treatment a good try for a reasonable period of time without success.

"We aim above the mark to hit the mark."
~Ralph Waldo Emerson

In the end, it may be that you do not get all the way to a cure, but you can still improve a great deal and experience much healing as a person.

How long to give your treatment options?

Any therapy could *begin* helping as quickly as within a few hours or days in a chronic condition. However, on average, you should be able to look back after six months and again after one year from when you set your intention and start your treatment program — especially the constitutional treatment — and realize that you have come a very long way. Nutritional supplements are not drugs and may require 4-6 months to begin hitting their maximum benefit, even if they start working sooner.

Five and ten years from now, you may look back and see that you have transformed or at least that you are in a wholly different place as a human being than you were at the worst of your chronic condition. In most cases, your healing process will have progressed noticeably.

Also, **expect that the improvements are lasting**, not that you are better one month and then back to where you started the next. If you get better and then relapse, the treatment is not acting at a sufficiently deep level of the system to hold. Discuss the situation with your providers and make adjustments in the overall plan. This may mean changing to another treatment option level or adding another type of care within a given level. It may also mean changing to another provider.

One approach that I like to use is applying major concepts from one field to another. Somehow deeper truths reveal themselves when you find the information pointing in the same direction. Thus, expand your reading beyond books on health and healing. For instance, a short little book like *The Dip* (see Resources), one that many business entrepreneurs might read, can help you frame your own progress with your health care choices in terms of when it makes sense for you to stay with a treatment or a provider and when to quit and move on to a different treatment or a different provider of a treatment for which you still hold hope of benefit. Another simple but profound book, *The Tipping Point*, might help you see how many factors converged to set you off onto a path of illness and how many other factors and changes might converge to re-direct you onto a good healing path.

Pacing

Your disease and your healing will have their own pace. You will find it necessary to honor that pace. Trying to rush it is counterproductive and will be another lesson to learn along the way. The pace of systemic healing usually reflects the intrinsic way you are in life – perhaps fast and intense or slow and methodical. **You heal in your own way just as you develop disease in your own way.**

"Adopt the pace of nature: her secret is patience."
~Ralph Waldo Emerson

What to Look For

In conventional (local, body part) medicine, the changes that you should expect are control of symptoms or problems in whatever local body part the treatment is targeting. Other changes are typically side effects, undesirable changes in other body parts such as indigestion or blurry vision or dizziness or headaches.

In whole systems care, the changes that you should expect are both general or global and local. Globally, your overall energy and sense of well-being should improve. In general, your dynamics as a system, your resilience or ability to bounce back from symptom flares, minor stressors, and major life events, should improve. With more resilience, the duration of symptom flares should become shorter and less severe in intensity. What shifts is the tendency to express the symptoms, rather than the momentary expression itself.

The patterning of the local symptoms that concerned you originally should become less frequent and/or less severe and perhaps even stop happening over time. Additional local symptoms that you had then, but had forgotten to mention in your initial evaluation, may also be lessened or gone.

Furthermore, you may have observed temporary re-emergence of old symptoms that you had forgotten for a while, old behaviors or old physical symptoms. Perhaps you came in for asthma, but then in the course of treatment you notice fewer and less severe asthma attacks but a return of diarrhea that you had many years before. Eventually the diarrhea will fade out, perhaps replaced for a while with a skin rash or an increased tendency to catch colds (a less severe form of disease than your chronic illness flares), which will itself gradually end with the passage of more time.

In short, the course of healing reveals the wisdom of the body as an intact indivisible system in shifting the manifestations of disease back in time, as though rewinding a stored memory in a tape program and in moving the manifestations from upper body to lower body and from more essential organs (heart, lung, kidneys) to less important organs (skin, mucous membranes). You, as a system, change how you live in your world.

In summary, you are an indivisible living network system that is currently manifesting a chronic disease. The most effective treatment for you is a system-oriented package of options that speak to your highest levels of organization as a system.

"There's no place like home...there's no place like home..."
~Dorothy Gale, *The Wizard of Oz*

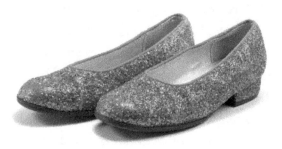

Figure 7-2

Epilogue

Now what?

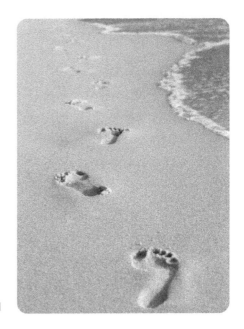

Figure E-1

"If you fall down seven times, get up eight."
~Chinese Proverb

So, now that you see the big picture, have chosen your preferred approaches to a personalized holistic health care plan, and understand how to evaluate your progress, what are your next specific steps?

Here is a brief To Do list to get you on your journey of healing. These are only suggestions – again, tailoring the program to your needs is what this book emphasizes. Health psychologists also know that doctors and patients can get paralyzed and take no action when faced with multiple choices. To sidestep decision paralysis, focus on the step-by-step process.

First Steps Action Plan:

1. Write out and review your current choices for treatment options. If you are not sure what to pick, educate yourself as a consumer with one of the resource books, audios, and DVDs listed at the back of this book.

2. Set your healing intention. Put it into words that you write down in a journal, as a screensaver or other reminder on your computer screen, and as an affirmation that you repeat silently or aloud to yourself daily just before you go to sleep.

3. Get more information on the constitutional level of care that you chose – both the therapy itself and the local, regional, and/or national practitioners who offer what you want. Possible ways to find a good practitioner include:

- Use word of mouth from family, friends, staff at other health care professionals' offices

- Look for small area newspapers or newsletters on holistic or alternative medicine with stories and ads about various providers

- Go on-line with web-browsing to search for official organization websites that list certified and/or licensed practitioners of a specific form of CAM. The Resources list at the back of this book gives you a start on some of the website URLs for these organizations.

4. Meet with your primary care provider and discuss your plans. Explain that you appreciate them and their treatment options, but you are thoughtfully exploring additional options. You want to work with them, openly, to find helpful answers to your health problems.

Many practitioners have ways to accommodate people who travel for their care. If you look for a practitioner who does "acupuncture," as an example, but you accept whoever is easiest to access — or even cheapest — you may not end up receiving the type of acupuncture best suited to your health care needs. Make sure to check carefully the credentials, training background, treatment philosophy, and current approaches to practice of each provider you consult. For basics such as professional misconduct, licensing boards in each state can provide information as to whether or not previous clients have lodged malpractice or ethical complaints against a given practitioner.

Research suggests that many users of alternative medicine in Western countries are financially able to afford paying out-of-pocket for the products and services they need for their health care. Increasingly, health care insurers are paying for a small number of alternative medicine services, *e.g.*, for a fixed numbers of visits.

But, what if you have limited resources to pay for holistic products and services? What if you live in a rural area, far from most holistic practitioners?

You can still get the help that you need. People who live in less affluent countries and/or low-income situations also use alternative medicine. If you look into your options, you will find that there will be ways to access help at low or even no cost within each of the levels of care described in this book. You may have to be a bit more innovative and flexible in designing and implementing your personal holistic health care plan, but you can do it.

In many cases, you can simply identify and choose options that are easily accessible to you at low or no cost. Low-cost books and internet websites can provide excellent information if you choose carefully. How do you know? Look for staying power in the field. People with solid credentials who have continued to speak and write books in a field for years are likely to offer the most reliable information available at the time than are the latest guru with no track record in the field. This is not to say that new faces and new ideas are all risky and to be avoided – far from it.

It is just that today's fad in alternative medicine often fades into the next and the next and the next. There is a wisdom to not necessarily being the first or the last adopter of an idea or treatment in holistic health, especially when research is so limited and/or hard to interpret for conflicting results in different studies (*i.e.*, when experts disagree). When convergent sources tell you that something might be helpful and your own experience tells you that it is good for you, then trust your judgment. Then, for safety, plan to re-evaluate each treatment choice regularly as new information comes up, not only outside yourself, but also within yourself in terms of how you feel and what you can do in your world.

If distance is an issue, emphasizing education and training in self-care methods will be invaluable. Once you have had a face-to-face meeting for your intake evaluations, you also can use telephone, internet-based phone and webcam options to get follow-up care involving less travel and expense, with many of your chosen providers who are located at a distance. Although skeptics may cringe at the suggestion, people who gravitate to subtle energy therapies will find that seasoned and experienced subtle energy healers also offer distance healing. They report that people can receive comparable benefits to those from in-person sessions, including help with severe chronic medical problems.

In other situations, you may be able to offer to trade or barter, in part or whole, your own products and services for those of practitioners whose help you need and want. Here is a sample personal holistic health care plan for a person of limited financial means and strong motivation to get on her healing journey (Table E-1). You can see that many of these suggestions are approaches for good self-care that anyone can consider including in a full holistic healing plan, whether or not they can access practitioners because of distance and/or financial challenges.

Table E-1

Sample personalized health care plan for a person with limited access and/or financial resources

LEVEL OF HEALTH CARE OPTIONS	Fill in Your Specific Choice (see Chapter 4)
1 Spiritual	Set the global healing intention: I am healthy and free to express my unique self in my world for the highest good. Pray, meditate, and/or repeat affirmations as suits your beliefs.
2 Constitutional	To reduce biochemical stress on the constitution: ❏ Self-care acupressure for acute pain, indigestion, etc. to reduce reliance on pain medications ❏ Low-cost, self-care homeopathic remedies for first aid and acute illnesses to reduce reliance on over-the-counter drugs

2a Subtle Energy	❑ Training in self-care qi gong (*e.g.*, Spring Forest type) ❑ Follow-up care as resources permit with an experienced distance healer for practitioner-provided care
3 Mind-Body	❑ Writing in journal regularly ❑ Making collages of images of healing ❑ Meditating and/or practicing yoga at home
4 Structural	❑ Use osteopathic self-care stretching exercises ❑ Get weekly massage from significant other or a friend with training in the fundamentals of massage
5 Preventive	❑ Practice good sleep hygiene ❑ Replace less health-promoting foods that foster inflammation or disease with better choices now available at reasonable cost at many supermarkets ❑ Take a walk at least three times per week
6 Biochemical/Biological	❑ Take a good multivitamin/multimineral supplement daily ❑ Add key nutritional supplement support, as affordable, from discount vitamin stores and during sales at large drugstore chains

In summary, you can get there from here. You need clarity from available information, expert advice and assistance where appropriate, courage, determination, support from other people, persistence, and, above all, a readiness to change out of bad ruts into good ones. Remember your ABC Principle for personalized holistic healing (Assess, Balance, Coordinate). Your journey and your story will be unique – sometimes painful, sometimes exhilarating – and, ultimately, rewarding.

"Begin at the beginning and go on till you come to the end; then stop."
~Lewis Carroll, Alice in Wonderland

Definitions

Constitutional or Whole-Person-System Approaches

Alternative whole medical systems are built upon complete systems of theory and practice. Each system includes a unique type of patient-provider therapeutic relationship and diagnostic process that differs from that in conventional medicine. All of these systems other than homeopathy also use multiple modalities in a coordinated treatment package to address the diagnosis of the problem within their conceptual framework or way of thinking. Even though homeopathy uses a single, individualized remedy for treating the overall pattern of constitutional disease, homeopaths also advise patients to give the remedy its best chance of helping by also removing any obstacles to cure, such as poor dietary and other lifestyle habits.

Often, these systems have evolved apart from and earlier than the conventional Western mainstream medical approach used in the United States. These systems see the person as a living system in which an invisible vital force or *qi* (subtle energy) moves.

Examples of alternative medical systems that have developed in Western cultures include homeopathic medicine (Germany) and naturopathic medicine (which combines multiple modalities such as nutrition, diet, homeopathy, botanicals (herbs)). Examples of systems that have developed in non-Western cultures include traditional Chinese medicine (China) and Ayurveda (India).

The ones that have the oldest traditions that focus on treating the person as a whole system — embedded within nature as the larger context — are homeopathic medicine, traditional Chinese medicine (which includes acupuncture), and Ayurveda. Naturopathic practice can draw on any or all of these other whole systems and may or may not apply the global versus the local mindset to treatment decisions.

Ayurveda ("ah-yur-VAY-dah") is a complementary and alternative medicine (CAM) alternative medical system that has been practiced primarily in the Indian subcontinent for 5,000 years. Ayurveda includes diet and herbal remedies and emphasizes the use of body, mind, and spirit in disease prevention and treatment.

Homeopathic medicine is a CAM alternative medical system. In homeopathic medicine, there is a belief that "like cures like," meaning that small, highly diluted and intensively shaken (succussed) quantities of medicinal substances made from animal, mineral, or plant origin are given to cure unique patterns of symptoms, when the same substances given at higher or more concentrated doses would actually cause the same pattern of symptoms. Medicines (remedies) are chosen as a similar match to the entire pattern of physical, emotional, and mental symptoms that a patient experiences. The homeopathic diagnosis and the treatment are the same – the person is seen as being in a particular state or pattern/rut in which symptoms are the manifestations of the same whole person disturbance showing up in various body parts. In successful homeopathic treatment, the remedy will shift the patient out of the rut into a healthier pattern of being and functioning at all levels in the world.

Traditional Chinese medicine (TCM) is the current name for an ancient system of health care from China. TCM is based on a concept of balanced *qi* (pronounced "chee"), or vital energy, that is believed to flow throughout the body. *Qi* is proposed to regulate a person's spiritual, emotional, mental, and physical balance and to be influenced by the opposing forces of yin (negative energy) and yang (positive energy). Disease is proposed to result from the flow of *qi* being disrupted and yin and yang becoming imbalanced. Among the components of TCM are herbal and nutritional therapy, restorative physical exercises (*e.g.*, tai chi), meditation, acupuncture, and remedial massage.

Acupuncture is a method of healing developed in China at least 2,000 years ago, and is usually part of traditional Chinese medicine. Today, acupuncture describes a family of procedures involving stimulation of specialized anatomical points (acupoints) on the body by a variety of techniques. Acupuncture practitioners believe that there is an interrelated energetic network connecting the acupuncture points and passing information very rapidly throughout the entire person (meridians).

American practices of acupuncture often incorporate medical traditions from China, Japan, Korea, and other countries. The acupuncture technique that has been most studied scientifically involves penetrating the skin with thin, solid, metallic needles that are manipulated by the hands or by electrical stimulation.

Subtle Energy Therapies. Energy therapies involve the use of subtle energy fields that extend outside around and into the physical body. Many practitioners of acupuncture and homeopathy consider those whole system interventions to exert their effects at least in part via shifting subtle energy fields.

In general, biofield therapies are intended to affect energy fields that purportedly surround and penetrate the human body. The existence of such fields has not yet been scientifically proven, although some measurements of light, sound, and magnetic fields suggest their existence. Some forms of energy therapy manipulate biofields by applying pressure and/or manipulating the body by placing the hands in, or through, these fields, but many of these therapies are done at a short or long distance from the body. Examples include *qi gong, Reiki, Johrei,* Therapeutic Touch, and Healing Touch.

Qi gong is a component of traditional Chinese medicine that combines movement, meditation, and regulation of breathing to enhance the flow of qi (an ancient term given to what is believed to be vital energy) in the body, improve blood circulation, and enhance immune function. People can use internal qi gong practices for self-care or receive treatment with external qi gong from a master practitioner.

Reiki is a Japanese word representing Universal Life Energy. *Reiki* is based on the belief that when spiritual energy is channeled through a *Reiki* practitioner, the patient's spirit is healed, which in turn heals the physical body.

Therapeutic Touch is derived from an ancient technique called laying-on of hands. It is based on the premise that it is the healing force of the therapist that affects the patient's recovery; healing is promoted when the body's energies are in balance; and, by passing their hands over the patient, healers can identify energy imbalances. *Healing Touch* is similar to Therapeutic Touch but has a more systematic training approach. Both Therapeutic Touch and Healing Touch arose within the professional RN nursing community, in which holism is considered a foundational concept.

This document does not address bioelectromagnetic-based therapies involve the unconventional use of readily measurable electromagnetic fields, such as pulsed fields, magnetic fields, or alternating-current or direct-current fields.

Mind-Body Interventions

Mind-body medicine uses a variety of techniques designed to enhance the mind's capacity to affect bodily function and symptoms. Some techniques that were considered CAM in the past have become mainstream (for example, patient support groups and cognitive-behavioral therapy). Other mind-body techniques are still considered CAM, including guided imagery, biofeedback, meditation, prayer, mental healing, and therapies that use creative outlets such as art, music, or dance.

Manipulative and Body-Based Methods

Manipulative and body-based methods in CAM are based on manipulation and/or movement of one or more parts of the body. Some examples include chiropractic or osteopathic manipulation, and massage.

Chiropractic is a CAM alternative medical system. It focuses on the relationship between bodily structure (primarily that of the spine) and function, and how that relationship affects the preservation and restoration of health. Chiropractors use manipulative therapy of the spine as an integral treatment tool.

Osteopathic medicine is a form of medicine that, in part, emphasizes diseases arising in the musculoskeletal system with a focus on soft tissue adjustment. There is an underlying belief that all of the body's systems work together, and disturbances in one system may affect function elsewhere in the body. Some osteopathic physicians practice osteopathic manipulation, a full-body system of hands-on techniques to alleviate pain, restore function, and promote health and well-being.

Massage therapists manipulate muscle and connective tissue to enhance function of those tissues and promote relaxation and well-being. Many types of manual-based therapies fall under the broad heading of massage but vary in their techniques. Some can be physically very intense (*e.g.*, Rolfing) and others more gentle (*e.g.*, Trager).

Biochemical/Biologically Based Therapies

Western pharmaceutically-based therapies in mainstream medicine use primarily highly purified synthetic drugs, though many drugs originated in natural substances such as herbs or other plants. Pharmaceutical drugs usually target specific physical or biochemical mechanisms within the physical body to oppose, block, change, or stimulate a local receptor for a particular cellular function. Examples are anti-histamines, anti-biotics, anti-depressants, or anti-hypertensives.

Some therapeutic agents in conventional medicine are just replacements for reduced or missing biochemical substances in the body such as insulin, a hormone normally produced by the pancreas (an issue for Type 1 diabetics), or dopamine, a brain chemical normally found in certain areas of the brain (an issue for people with Parkinson's disease).

Biologically based therapies in CAM use substances found in nature, such as herbs, foods, and vitamins. Some examples include dietary supplements, herbal products, and the use of other so-called natural but controversial therapies (for example, using shark cartilage to treat cancer). Many people who use CAM use botanical products such as Echinacea, St. John's Wort, Ginseng, or Gingko biloba. In such products, the whole herb is involved rather than isolating and purifying one specific chemical constitutent from the whole mixture (the Western mainstream way of identifying therapeutic agents).

Dietary supplements. Congress defined the term "dietary supplement" in the Dietary Supplement Health and Education Act (DSHEA) of 1994. A dietary supplement is a product (other than tobacco) taken by mouth that contains a "dietary ingredient" intended to supplement the diet. Dietary ingredients may include vitamins, minerals, herbs or other botanicals, amino acids, and substances such as enzymes, organ tissues, and metabolites. Dietary supplements come in many forms, including extracts, concentrates, tablets, capsules, gel caps, liquids, and powders. They have special requirements for labeling. Under DSHEA, dietary supplements are considered foods, not drugs.

Note: Naturopathic medicine, or naturopathy, is a CAM alternative medical system. Naturopathic medicine straddles mindsets in health care. Philosophically, naturopathy is similar to homeopathy, Chinese medicine, and Ayurveda in that it proposes that there is a healing power or vital life force in the body that establishes, maintains, and restores health. Practitioners work with the patient with a goal of supporting this power, through treatments such as nutrition and lifestyle counseling, dietary supplements, medicinal plants, exercise, homeopathy, and treatments from traditional Chinese medicine.

In practice, naturopaths have licenses to prescribe pharmaceutical drugs in some States, and some naturopaths simply substitute natural products for pharmaceutical drugs when they can, with a focus on "fixing" a problem at the local body part level. It requires discussion with each practitioner to determine how he/she uses drugs and naturopathic therapies.

(Adapted from public domain source:
http://nccam.nih.gov/health/)

Resources

Track Down Whom and What You Need

Websites, Books, and Other Sources to Enrich
Creating Your Own Treatment Program

> *"Whatever you can do, or dream you can, begin it.*
> *Boldness has genius, power, and magic in it."*
> ~Johann Wolfgang von Goethe

The resources listed below give you a way to learn more about your options and to find sources of assistance in your healing process. The author cannot assure the reader that recommendations, providers, or treatments encountered in pursuing these resources all will be in agreement with the opinions, perspectives, or information expressed in this book. Nevertheless, these offer a valuable starting point for your explorations using the framework outlined here.

Choosing a CAM Practitioner

U.S. National Institutes of Health:
http://nccam.nih.gov/health/practitioner/index.htm

Different practitioners may use therapies with the same name (even if they are calling them complementary and alternative medicine) in either Western conventional mindset or whole person systemic mindset ways. It is up to you as the health care consumer to discuss what you want with your providers. Know not only what treatments you receive, but also how the provider uses them in your case.

Working with your Conventional Physician

MedicineNet network of Board-certified physicians and allied health professionals:
http://www.medicinenet.com

See their downloadable reports on

- "How to help your doctor"
  http://www.medicinenet.com/script/main/art.asp?articlekey=23815

- "Popular medications and information you should know"
  http://www.medicinenet.com/pdf/popularmedicationsguide.pdf

Health and Life Coaching

Some health coaches advise people with chronic diseases in coping better with the everyday life challenges that arise.

Here are some useful links:

- www.davidsperorn.com
- www.healingwell.com
- www.holistic.com

Some life coaches advise people with and without chronic disease on taking stock of their personal Big Picture and moving forward in their overall lives in a positive way. Do some research to see if a particular coach's area of expertise and approach meet your unique needs. Here are some useful links:

- www.coach-federation.org
- www.expansiveliving.com
- www.intuitivelifecoaching.com

Other General Health and Disease Information Websites

- www.webmd.com
- www.medifocus.com
- www.cdc.gov (including website on preventing chronic disease: http://www.cdc.gov/nccdphp/)
- http://health.nih.gov/

Information and Assessment Sources on Whole Person Healing

- www.holisticmedicine.org (American Holistic Medical Association)

- www.naturopathic.org (American Association of Naturopathic Physicians)

- www.ahna.org/home/home.html (American Holistic Nurses Association)

- www.drweil.com

- www.healthy.net

- www.wellpeople.com

Overview Books on Treatment Options

Castleman M. *Blended Medicine: The Best Choices in Healing.* Rodale, 2000.

Goldberg B. ed. *Alternative Medicine: The Definitive Guide.* 2nd ed., 2002.

Pelletier K. ed. *New Medicine. Complete Family Health Guide.* DK Adult, 2007.

Travis JW, Ryan RS. *Wellness Workbook. How to Achieve Enduring Health and Vitality.* 3rd ed. Celestial Arts, 2004.

Weil A. *Natural Health, Natural Medicine: The Complete Guide to Wellness and Self-Care for Optimum Health.* Houghton Mifflin, 2004.

Setting Healing Intention

Dyer WW. *The Power of Intention. Learning to Co-create Your World Your Way.* Carlsbad, CA: Hay House, 2004.

Vitale J. *The Attractor Factor: 5 Easy Steps for Creating Wealth (or Anything Else) from the Inside Out.* John Wiley, 2005

Dossey L. *Healing Words.* Harper San Francisco, 1997.

Dossey L. *Be Careful What You Pray For...You Just Might Get It.* Harper San Francisco, 1998.

Chopra D. *The Book of Secrets: Unlocking the Hidden Dimensions of Your Life.* Harmony, 2004.

Constitutional Treatment Options
Chinese Medicine

National Certification Commission for Acupuncture and Oriental Medicine:
http://dol.jkmcomm.com/acupuncture/default.asp

Cohen MJ. *The Chinese Way to Healing: Many Paths to Wholeness.* NY: Berkley Publishing, 1996.

Connelly DM. *Traditional Acupuncture: The Law of the Five Elements.* Traditional Acupuncture Institute Inc., 1994

Kaptchuk T. *The Web that Has No Weaver: Understanding Chinese Medicine.* McGraw-Hill, 2000.

Classical Homeopathy

National Center for Homeopathy:
http://nationalcenterforhomeopathy.org/

Cummings S, Ullman D. *Everybody's Guide to Homeopathic Medicines.* Jeremy Tarcher/Putnam, 2004.

Lansky A. RL. *Impossible Cure: The Promise of Homeopathy.* RL Ranch, 2003.

Jonas WB, Jacobs J. *Healing with Homeopathy: The Doctors' Guide.* Warner Books, 1998.

Ullman D. *The Homeopathic Revolution. Why Famous People and Cultural Heroes Choose Homeopathy.* North Atlantic Books, 2007.

Ayurvedic Healing

The Ayurvedic Institute (New Mexico):
http://www.ayurveda.com/index.html

Chopra D. *Perfect Health: The Complete Mind/Body Guide (revised).* Harmony, 2001.

Krishan S. *Essential Ayurveda: What It Is and What It Can Do for You.* Novato, CA: New World Library, 2003

Frawley D. *Ayurvedic Healing: A Comprehensive Guide* 2nd ed., Lotus Press, 2000.

Subtle Energy Treatment Options

See Goldberg B. ed. *Alternative Medicine: The Definitive Guide.* 2nd ed., 2002.

Gerber R. *A Practical Guide to Vibrational Medicine: Energy Healing and Spiritual Transformation.* Harper, 2001.

Hover-Kramer D. *Healing Touch: A Guide Book for Practitioners,* 2nd edition. Cengage Delmar Learning, 2001.

Krieger D. *Accepting Your Power to Heal: The Personal Practice of Therapeutic Touch.* Bear and Co., 1993.

Lin C, Rebstock G. *Born a Healer.* Spring Forest *Qi Gong* Company, 2003.

Lin C. *Spring Forest Qigong Course* (Book, Audio tapes, VHS & CD). Minnetonka, MN: Learning Strategies Corp., 2000.

Rand WL. *The Reiki Touch: complete home learning system.* Sounds True, 2005.

Mind-Body Treatment Options

Borysenko J. *Minding the Body, Mending the Mind (revised).* Da Capo Lifelong Books, 2007.

Rossman M. *Guided Imagery for Self-Healing: An Essential Resource for Anyone Seeking Wellness.* 2nd ed. HJ Kramer, 2000

Bouton E. *Journaling from the Heart.* Whole Heart Publications, 2000.

Davis M et al. *The Relaxation & Stress Reduction Workbook.* 5th ed. New Harbinger, 2000.

Gurgevich S. *The Self-Hypnosis Home Study Course* (boxed set – multimedia). Sounds True Publishers, 2005.

Affirmware Sculptor 3 software (http://affirmwaresculptor3.info/). Integrates seven technologies to use at your computer 10 minutes a day – helps you create your own affirmations and support them with advanced multisensory inputs.

Best of Stress Management (http://www.bio-medical.com/) – a 10-week Home study Multimedia Course to develop your own relaxation program

The Sleep Advisor (http://thesleepadvisor.com/) – a software program by a sleep disorders specialist to help you evaluate your sleep problems and find non-pharmacological options.

Sound Medicine: Music for Healing – Steven Halpern Relaxation Audio CD, 2002.

Structural/Manual Manipulation Treatment Options

See Goldberg B. ed. *Alternative Medicine: The Definitive Guide.* 2nd ed., 2002.

American College of Osteopathic Family Physicians. *Somatic Dysfunction in Osteopathic Family Medicine.* Lippincott, Williams, and Wilkins, 2006.

Forem J. *Healing Yourself with Pressure Point Therapy: Simple, Effective Techniques for Massaging Away More Than 100 Annoying Ailments.* Prentice Hall, 1999.

Gevitz N. *The DOs: Osteopathic Medicine in America.* Johns Hopkins University Press, 2004.

Lidell L, et al. *The Book Of Massage: The Complete Step by Step Guide To Eastern And Western Technique.* Fireside, 2001.

Reizer JL. *Chiropractic Made Simple: Working With the Controlling Laws of Nature.* Pagefree Publishing, 2002.

Preventive Medicine Options

See Goldberg B. ed. *Alternative Medicine: The Definitive Guide.* 2nd ed., 2002.

Benson H, Stuart E. *Wellness Book: The Comprehensive Guide to Maintaining Health and Treating Stress-Related Illness.* Scribner, 1993.

Luskin F, Pelletier K. *Stress Free for Good : 10 Scientifically Proven Life Skills for Health and Happiness.* Harper San Francisco, 2005.

Weil, A. *Eight Weeks to Optimum Health, Revised Edition: A Proven Program for Taking Full Advantage of Your Body's Natural Healing Power.* Knopf, 2006.

Physical/Biochemical Treatment Options

Pizzorno J. *Total Wellness : Improve Your Health by Understanding the Body's Healing Systems.* Prima Lifestyles 1996.

Galland L. *Power Healing : Use the New Integrated Medicine to Cure Yourself.* Random House, 1998.

Thiel RJ. *Combining Old and New : Naturopathy for the 21st Century.* Whitman Publications, 2001.

Self-Help Books on Coping with Chronic Disease

Bouvard M. *Healing: A Life with Chronic Illness.* UPNE, 2007.

Lorig K, Holman H, Sobel D, Laurent D, Minor M. *Living a Healthy Life with Chronic Conditions. Self-Management of Heart Disease, Fatigue, Arthritis, Worry Diabetes, Frustration, Asthma, Pain, Emphysema, and Others (3rd edition).* Bull Publishing, 2006.

Salvucci P. *Self-Care Now! 30 Tips to Help You Take Care of Yourself When Chronic Illness Turns Your Life Upside Down.* P Salvucci, 2001.

Spero D. *The Art of Getting Well: Maximizing Health and Well-being When You Have a Chronic Illness.* Alameda, CA: Hunter House, 2002.

Wells SM. *A Delicate Balance. Living Successfully with Chronic Illness.* Cambridge, MA: Perseus, 2000.

The Nature of Healing

Hirshberg C. *Remarkable Recovery. What Extraordinary Healings Teach Us about Getting Well and Staying Well.* Riverhead, 1996.

Chopra D. *Quantum Healing: Exploring the Frontiers of Mind/Body Medicine.* Bantam, 1990.

Lerner M. *Choices in Healing: Integrating the Best of Conventional and Complementary Approaches to Cancer.* MIT Press, 1996.

Moyers B. *Healing and the Mind.* Doubleday, 1995.

Remen, RN. *Kitchen Table Wisdom. Stories that Heal.* Riverhead, 2006/1997.

Weil A. *Spontaneous Healing : How to Discover and Embrace Your Body's Natural Ability to Maintain and Heal Itself.* Ballantine, 2000.

Weil A. *Health and Healing: The Philosophy of Integrative Medicine and Optimum Health.* Houghton Mifflin, 2004.

Miller, W, C'debaca J. *Quantum Change: When Epiphanies and Sudden Insights Transform Ordinary Lives.* Guilford, 2001.

Big Picture Idea Books on Relevant Concepts to Apply to Personalized Holistic Health Care
(for Understanding Illness as a Process, Individualizing Care, and Optimizing Coping with the Process of Healing)

Gladwell, M. *The Tipping Point. How Little Things Can Make a Big Difference.* Little, Brown, 2000.

Godin, S. *The Dip: A Little Book That Teaches You When to Quit (and When to Stick).* Portfolio, 2007.

Penn M. *Microtrends: The Small Forces Behind Tomorrow's Big Changes.* Twelve, 2007.

General Information on the Nature of Complex Systems and Networks

Barabasi AL. *Linked. How everything is connected to everything else and what it means for business, science, and everyday life.* Cambridge, MA: Plume; 2003.

Bar-Yam Y. *Making Things Work: Solving Complex Problems in a Complex World.* NECSI Knowledge Press, 2004.

Buchanan M. *Nexus: Small Worlds and the Groundbreaking Science of Networks.* WW Norton, 2002.

Gleick J. *Chaos: Making a New Science.* Penguin Books, 1987.

Kauffman S. *At Home in the Universe: The Search for the Laws of Self-Organization and Complexity.* Oxford University Press, 1996.

Laszlo E. *The Systems View of the World. A Holistic Vision for Our Time*. Hampton Press, 1996 (4th printing 2002).

Lewin R. *Complexity: Life at the Edge of Chaos.* 2nd ed. University of Chicago Press, 2000

Strogatz S. *Sync: The Emerging Science of Spontaneous Order*. Hyperion, 2003.

Waldrop MM. *Complexity: The Emerging Science at the Edge of Order and Chaos*. Simon and Schuster, 1992.

Watts DJ. *Six Degrees: The Science of a Connected Age*. WW Norton, 2003.

West BJ. *Where Medicine Went Wrong: Rediscovering the Path to Complexity*. World Scientific, 2006.

Beyond Complex Systems

Byrne R. *The Secret*. Atria Books, 2006.

McTaggart L. *The Field: The Quest for the Secret Force of the Universe*. Harper, 2003.

Talbot M. *The Holographic Universe*. Harper, 1992.

Tolle, E. *A New Earth. Awakening to Your Life's Purpose*. Plume, 2006.

Background Research Readings

Note: The purpose of these selected research articles on both theory and clinical studies is to illustrate major themes discussed in this book for advanced readers.

Concepts include

(a) using complex, coordinated treatment packages as whole systems of care rather than single interventions; and

(b) focusing on person-centered individualized care and whole-person outcomes.

The background research article list is not intended to provide a comprehensive database of studies testing treatment efficacy of each specific CAM treatment for each specific chronic disease diagnosis. For updated information regarding the latest research findings on single interventions for specific conventional medical diagnoses, consumers should search http://www.pubmed.com and/or http://www.nccam.nih.gov.

Ahn AC, Tewari M, Poon CS, Phillips RS. The limits of reductionism in medicine: could systems biology offer an alternative? *PLoS Med.* 2006; 3 (6):e208.

Alraek T, Baerheim, A. The effect of prophylactic acupuncture treatment in women with recurrent cystitis: kidney patients fare better. *Journal of Alternative & Complementary Medicine* 2003; 9 (5):651-8.

Almeras L, Eyles D, Benech P, Laffite D, Villard C, Patatian A, Boucraut J, Mackay-Sim A, McGrath J, Féron F. Developmental vitamin D deficiency alters brain protein expression in the adult rat: implications for neuropsychiatric disorders. *Proteomics* 2007; 7 (5):769-80.

Altindag O, Celik H. Total antioxidant capacity and the severity of the pain in patients with fibromyalgia. *Redox Report* 2006; 11 (3):131-5.

Bai L, Tian J, Qin W, Pan X, Yang L, Chen P, Chen H, Dai J, Ai L, Zhao B. Exploratory analysis of functional connectivity network in acupuncture study by a graph theory mode. *Conf Proc IEEE Eng Med Biol Soc* 2007; 1:2023-6.

Balon R. Mood, anxiety, and physical illness: body and mind, or mind and body? *Depression & Anxiety.* 2006; 23 (6):377-87.

Barabasi AL, Bonabeau E. Scale-free networks. *Scientific American.* 2003; 288 (5):60-9.

Barabasz A, Barabasz M. Effects of tailored and manualized hypnotic inductions for complicated irritable bowel syndrome patients. *Int J Clin Exp Hypn.* 2006; 54 (1):100-12.

Barnes PM, Powell-Griner E, McFann K et al. Complementary and alternative medicine use among adults: United States, 2002. Hyattsville, MD: National Center for Health Statistics.

Barringer TA, Kirk JK, Santaniello AC, Foley KL, Michielutte R. Effect of a multivitamin and mineral supplement on infection and quality of life. A randomized, double-blind, placebo-controlled trial. *Annals of Internal Medicine* 2003; 138 (5):365-71.

Bell IR, Caspi O, Schwartz GE et al. Integrative medicine and systemic outcomes research: issues in the emergence of a new model for primary health care. *Archives of Internal Medicine.* 2002; 162 (2):133-40.

Bell IR, Koithan M. Models for the study of whole systems. *Integrative Cancer Therapies* 2006; 5 (4):293-307.

Bell IR, Lewis DA, 2nd, Brooks AJ et al. Individual differences in response to randomly assigned active individualized homeopathic and placebo treatment in fibromyalgia: implications of a double-blinded optional crossover design. *Journal of Alternative & Complementary Medicine* 2004a; 10 (2):269-83.

Bell IR, Lewis DA, 2nd, Schwartz GE et al. Electroencephalographic cordance patterns distinguish exceptional clinical responders with fibromyalgia to individualized homeopathic medicines. *Journal of Alternative & Complementary Medicine* 2004b; 10 (2):285-99.

Bensoussan A, Talley NJ, Hing M et al. Treatment of irritable bowel syndrome with Chinese herbal medicine: a randomized controlled trial. *JAMA* 1998; 280 (18):1585-9.

Block G, Jensen CD, Norkus EP, Dalvi TB, Wong LG, McManus JF, Hudes ML. Usage patterns, health, and nutritional status of long-term multiple dietary supplement users: a cross-sectional study. *Nutrition Journal.* 2007; 6 epub (1):30.

Bornhoft G, Wolf U, Ammon K et al. Effectiveness, safety and cost-effectiveness of homeopathy in general practice - summarized health technology assessment. *Forsch Komplementarmed* 2006; 13 Suppl 2:19-29.

Breuer GS, Orbach H, Elkayam O, Berkun Y, Paran D, Mates M, Nesher G. Perceived efficacy among patients of various methods of complementary alternative medicine for rheumatologic diseases. *Clinical Experimental Rheumatology.* 2005; 23 (5):693-6.

Cabyoglu MT, Ergene N, Tan U. The mechanism of acupuncture and clinical applications. International Journal of Neuroscience 2006; 116 (2):115-25.

Caspi O, Bell IR. One size does not fit all: aptitude-treatment interaction (ATI) as a conceptual framework for outcome research. Part I. What is ATI research? *Journal of Alternative & Complementary Medicine* 2004a; 10 (3):580-6.

Caspi O, Bell IR. One size does not fit all: aptitude-treatment interaction (ATI) as a conceptual framework for outcome research. Part II. Research designs and their application.

Journal of Alternative and Complementary Medicine. 2004b; 10 (4):698-705.

Cassileth BR, Deng GE, Gomez JE, Johnstone PA, Kumar N, Vickers AJ; American College of Chest Physicians. Complementary therapies and integrative oncology in lung cancer: ACCP evidence-based clinical practice guidelines (2nd edition). *Chest* 2007; 132 (3 Suppl):340S-54S.

Cassileth B, Trevisan C, Gubili J. Complementary therapies for cancer pain. *Current Pain Headache Report.* 2007; 11 (4):265-9.

Chou R, Huffman LH; American Pain Society; American College of Physicians. Nonpharmacologic therapies for acute and chronic low back pain: a review of the evidence for an American Pain Society/American College of Physicians clinical practice guideline. *Annals of Internal Medicine.* 2007; 147 (7):492-504.

Clayton AH, West SG. Combination therapy in fibromyalgia. *Current Pharm Des.* 2006; 12 (1):11-6.

Council JR, Kirsch I, Hafner LP. Expectancy versus absorption in the prediction of hypnotic responding. *Journal of Personality & Social Psychology* 1986; 50 (1):182-9.

Efferth T, Li PC, Konkimalla VS, Kaina B. From traditional Chinese medicine to rational cancer therapy. *Trends Molecular Medicine.* 2007; 13 (8):353-61.

Egger J, Carter CH, Soothill JF et al. Effect of diet treatment on enuresis in children with migraine or hyperkinetic behavior. *Clinical Pediatrics* 1992a; 31 (5):302-7.

Egger J, Carter CM, Graham PJ et al. Controlled trial of oligoantigenic treatment in the hyperkinetic syndrome. *Lancet* 1985; 1 (8428):540-5.

Egger J, Carter CM, Soothill JF et al. Oligoantigenic diet treatment of children with epilepsy and migraine. *Journal of Pediatrics* 1989; 114 (1):51-8.

Egger J, Carter CM, Wilson J, Turner MW, Soothill JF. Is migraine food allergy? A double-blind controlled trial of oligoantigenic diet treatment. *Lancet.* 1983; 2 (8355):865-9.

Egger J, Stolla A, McEwen LM. Controlled trial of hyposensitisation in children with food-induced hyperkinetic syndrome. *Lancet* 1992b; 339 (8802):1150-3.

Elder C, Aickin M, Bauer V, Cairns J, Vuckovic N. Randomized trial of a whole-system ayurvedic protocol for type 2 diabetes. *Alternative Therapies in Health & Medicine.* 2006; 12 (5):24-30.

Endres HG DH, Molsberger A. Role of acupuncture in the treatment of migraine. *Expert Reviews Neurother.* 2007; 7 (9):1121-34.

Fox RA, Joffres MR, Sampalli T, Casey J. The impact of a multi-disciplinary, holistic approach to management of patients diagnosed with multiple chemical sensitivity on health care utilization costs: an observational study. *Journal of Alternative & Complementary Medicine* 2007; 13 (2):223-9.

Frass M, Linkesch M, Banyai S et al. Adjunctive homeopathic treatment in patients with severe sepsis: a randomized, double-blind, placebo-controlled trial in an intensive care unit. *Homeopathy: the Journal of the Faculty of Homeopathy* 2005; 94 (2):75-80.

Fredrickson BL, Losada MF. Positive affect and the complex dynamics of human flourishing. *American Psychologist* 2005; 60 (7):678-86.

Frei H, Everts R, von Ammon K et al. Randomised controlled trials of homeopathy in hyperactive children: treatment procedure leads to an unconventional study design Experience with open-label homeopathic treatment preceding the Swiss ADHD placebo controlled, randomised, double-blind, cross-over trial. *Homeopathy: the Journal of the Faculty of Homeopathy* 2007; 96 (1):35-41.

Frei H, Everts R, von Ammon K, Kaufmann F, Walther D, Hsu-Schmitz SF, Collenberg M, Fuhrer K, Hassink R, Steinlin M, Thurneysen A. Homeopathic treatment of children with attention deficit hyperactivity disorder: a randomised, double blind, placebo controlled crossover trial. *European Journal of Pediatrics* 2005; 164 (12):758-67.

Gaede P, Pedersen, O. Multi-targeted and aggressive treatment of patients with type 2 diabetes at high risk: what are we waiting for? *Hormone Metabolism Research.* 2005; 37 (Suppl 1):76-82.

Gibson PR, Elms ANM, Ruding LA. Perceived treatment efficacy for conventional and alternative therapies reported by persons with multiple chemical sensitivity. *Environmental Health Perspectives* 2003; 111:1498-504.

Gupta N, Khera S, Vempati RP, Sharma R, Bijlani RL. Effect of yoga based lifestyle intervention on state and trait anxiety. *Indian Journal of Physiology & Pharmacology.* 2006; 50 (1):41-7.

Guthlin C, Lange O, Walach H. Measuring the effects of acupuncture and homoeopathy in general practice: an uncontrolled prospective documentation approach. *BMC Public Health* 2004; 4 (1):4.

Herman WH, Hoerger TJ, Brandle M et al. The cost-effectiveness of lifestyle modification or metformin in preventing type 2 diabetes in adults with impaired glucose tolerance. *Annals of Internal Medicine* 2005; 142 (5):323-32.

Heyland DK, Dodek P, Muscedere J, Day A, Cook D; for the Canadian Critical Care Trials Group. Randomized trial of combination versus monotherapy for the empiric treatment of suspected ventilator-associated pneumonia. *Critical Care Medicine* 2007; 12 (epub).

Honda K, Jacobson JS. Use of complementary and alternative medicine among United States adults: the influences of personality, coping strategies, and social support. *Preventive Medicine* 2005; 40 (1):46-53.

Hsiu H, Huang SM, Chao PT, Jan MY, Hsu TL, Wang WK, Wang YY. Microcirculatory characteristics of acupuncture points obtained by laser Doppler flowmetry. *Physiol Meas* 2007; 28 (10):N77-86.

Hui KK, Liu J, Makris N, Gollub RL, Chen AJ, Moore CI, Kennedy DN, Rosen BR, Kwong KK. Acupuncture modulates the limbic system and subcortical gray structures of the human brain: evidence from fMRI studies in normal subjects. *Human Brain Mapping* 2000; 9 (1):13-25.

Hui KK NE, Vangel MG, Liu J, Marina O, Napadow V, Hodge SM, Rosen BR, Makris N, Kennedy DN. Characterization of the "Deqi" Response in Acupuncture. *BMC Complementary & Alternative Medicine* 2007; 7 (1):33.

Husted C, Dhondup L. Tibetan Medical Interpretation of Myelin and Multiple Sclerosis. *Annals New York Academy Sciences* 2007; in press.

Keith CT, Borisy AA, Stockwell BR. Multicomponent therapeutics for networked systems. *Nature Reviews. Drug Discovery* 2005; 4 (1):71-8.

Kiecolt-Glaser JK, McGuire L, Robles TF et al. Psychoneuroimmunology and psychosomatic medicine: back to the future. *Psychosomatic Medicine* 2002; 64 (1):15-28.

Koithan M, Verhoef, M., Bell, I.R., Ritenbaugh, C., White, M., Mulkins, A. The process of whole person healing: "unstuckness" and beyond. *Journal of Alternative & Complementary Medicine* 2007; 13 (6):659-68.

Lang E, Liebig K, Kastner S, Neundörfer B, Heuschmann P. Multidisciplinary rehabilitation versus usual care for chronic low back pain in the community: effects on quality of life. *Spine J.* 2003; 3 (4):270-6.

Linde K, Streng A, Hoppe A, Weidenhammer W, Wagenpfeil S, Melchart D. Randomized trial vs. observational study of acupuncture for migraine found that patient characteristics differed but outcomes were similar. *Journal of Clinical Epidemiology* 2007; 60 (3):280-7.

Linden W, Moseley JV. The efficacy of behavioral treatments for hypertension. *Applied Psychophysiology & Biofeedback.* 2006; 31 (1):51-63.

Lipsitz LA, Goldberger, A.L. Loss of 'complexity' and aging. Potential applications of fractals and chaos theory to senescence. *JAMA* 1992; 267:1806-9.

Manheimer E, Linde K, Lao L, Bouter LM, Berman BM. Meta-analysis: acupuncture for osteoarthritis of the knee. *Annals of Internal Medicine* 2007; 146 (12):868-77.

Marlin RG, Anchel H, Gibson JC et al. An evaluation of multidisciplinary intervention for chronic fatigue syndrome with long-term follow-up, and a comparison with untreated controls. *American Journal of Medicine* 1998; 105 (3A):110S-4S.

Masi AT, White KP, Pilcher JJ. Person-centered approach to care, teaching, and research in fibromyalgia syndrome: justification from biopsychosocial perspectives in populations. *Seminars in Arthritis & Rheumatism.* 2002; 32 (2):71-93.

Maxion-Bergemann S, Wolf M, Bornhoft G et al. Complementary and alternative medicine costs - a systematic literature review. *Forsch Komplementarmed.* 2006; 13 (Suppl 2):42-5.

Morris CR, Bowen L, Morris AJ. Integrative therapy for fibromyalgia: possible strategies for an individualized treatment program. *Southern Medical Journal* 2005; 98 (2):177-84.

Narimanian M, Badalyan M, Panosyan V, Gabrielyan E, Panossian A, Wikman G, Wagner H. Randomized trial of a fixed combination (KanJang) of herbal extracts containing Adhatoda vasica, Echinacea purpurea and Eleutherococcus senticosus in patients with upper respiratory tract infections. *Phytomedicine* 2005; 12 (8):539-47.

Neff DF, Blanchard, E.B., Andrasik, F. The relationship between capacity for absorption and chronic headache patients' response to relaxation and biofeedback treatment. *Biofeedback & Self Regulation* 1983; 8 (1):177-83.

O'Connell KA, Skevington SM. To measure or not to measure? Reviewing the assessment of spirituality and religion in health-related quality of life. *Chronic Illness* 2007; 3 (1):77-87.

Owens JE, Taylor AG, Degood D. Complementary and alternative medicine and psychologic factors: toward an individual differences model of complementary and alternative medicine use and outcomes. *Journal of Alternative & Complementary Medicine* 1999; 5 (6):529-41.

Riley D, Fischer M, Singh B et al. Homeopathy and conventional medicine: an outcomes study comparing effectiveness in a primary care setting. *Journal of Alternative & Complementary Medicine* 2001; 7 (2):149-59.

Ritenbaugh C, Verhoef M, Fleishman S et al. Whole systems research: a discipline for studying complementary and alternative medicine. *Alternative Therapies in Health & Medicine* 2003; 9 (4):32-6.

Robinson N, Donaldson J, Watt H. Auditing outcomes and costs of integrated complementary medicine provision—the importance of length of follow up. *Complementary Therapies in Clinical Practice* 2006; 12 (4):249-57.

Schoenthaler SJ, Bier ID, Young K, Nichols D, Jansenns S. The effect of vitamin-mineral supplementation on the intelligence of American schoolchildren: a randomized, double-blind placebo-controlled trial. *Journal of Alternative & Complementary Medicine* 2000; 6 (1):19-29.

Siedentopf CM, Golaszewski SM, Mottaghy FM, Ruff CC, Felber S, Schlager A. Functional magnetic resonance imaging detects activation of the visual association cortex during laser acupuncture of the foot in humans. *Neuroscience Letters* 2002; 327 (1):53-6.

Steffek BD, Blanchard EB. The role of absorption capacity in thermal biofeedback treatment of vascular headache. *Biofeedback & Self Regulation* 1991; 16 (3):267-75.

Thomas KJ, MacPherson H, Ratcliffe J, Thorpe L, Brazier J, Campbell M, Fitter M, Roman M, Walters S, Nicholl JP. Longer term clinical and economic benefits of offering acupuncture care to patients with chronic low back pain. *Health Technology Assessment* 2005 Aug;9(32) 2005; 32 (iii-iv, ix-x):1-109.

Turk DC. The potential of treatment matching for subgroups of patients with chronic pain: lumping versus splitting. *Clinical Journal of Pain* 2005; 21 (1):44-55.

van Wassenhoven M, Ives G. An observational study of patients receiving homeopathic treatment. *Homeopathy* 2004; 93 (1):3-11.

Verhoef M, Lewith G, Ritenbaugh C et al. Whole systems research: moving forward. *Focus on Alternative and Complementary Therapies* 2004; 9 (2):87-90.

Verhoef MJ, Lewith G, Ritenbaugh C et al. Complementary and alternative medicine whole systems research: Beyond identification of inadequacies of the RCT. *Complementary Therapies in Medicine* 2005; 13 (3):206-12.

Ward NC, Hodgson JM, Croft KD, Burke V, Beilin LJ, IB. The combination of vitamin C and grape-seed polyphenols increases blood pressure: a randomized, double-blind, placebo-controlled trial. *Journal of Hypertension* 2005; 23 (2):427-34.

Weidenhammer W, Linde K, Streng A, Hoppe A, Melchart D. Acupuncture for chronic low back pain in routine care: a multicenter observational study. *Clinical Journal Pain.* 2007; 23 (2):128-35.

Witt C, Keil T, Selim D et al. Outcome and costs of homoeopathic and conventional treatment strategies: a comparative cohort study in patients with chronic disorders. *Complementary Therapies in Medicine* 2005; 13 (2):79-86.

Woolhouse M. Migraine and tension headache—a complementary and alternative medicine approach. *Aust Family Physician*. 2005; 34 (8):647-51.

Yao R. The thoughts and methods for clinical research on acupuncture treatment of chronic fatigue syndrome. *Journal of Traditional Chinese Medicine* 2007; 27 (3):163-5.

Yin C, Seo B, Park HJ, Cho M, Jung W, Choue R, Kim C, Park HK, Lee H, Koh H. Acupuncture, a promising adjunctive therapy for essential hypertension: a double-blind, randomized, controlled trial. *Neurology Research* 2007; 29 (Suppl 1):S98-S103.

Zhang GJ, Shi ZY, Liu S, Gong SH, Liu JQ, Liu JS. Clinical observation on treatment of depression by electro-acupuncture combined with paroxetine. *Chinese Journal of Integrative Medicine* 2007; 13 (3):228-30.

Illustration Credits

Front cover & Chap. breaks
  ABC Apples by Paul Kline
  www.istockphoto.com, 3289230, used with license.

I-1
  An Apple a Day Keeps the Doctor Away by Travis Manley
  www.dreamstime.com, 1982551, used with license.

Fig. 1-1
  Countryside walk by Matt Collingwood
  www.dreamstime.com, 188068, used with license.

Fig. 2-1
  Digital abstract by Emrah Turudu
  www.istockphoto.com, 2160078, used with license.

Fig. 2-2A
  Auto mechanic by Caraman
  www.dreamstime.com, 33888, used with license.

Fig. 2.2B
> Jump at sunrise by Elena Pokrovskaya
> www.dreamstime.com, 2503514, used with license.

Fig. 2.3
> Levels of systems by Iris Bell
> www.irisbell.com

Fig. 2-4A
> The magic wood by Valentin Mosichev
> www.dreamstime.com, 239169, used with license.

Fig. 2-4B
> Lonely tree silhouhette by Cristian Nitu
> www.dreamstime.com, 217549, used with license.

Fig. 2-4C
> Pine tree branch with single cone by Ivan Chuyev
> www.dreamstime.com, 256924, used with license.

Fig. 2-5A
> Low performance business team dynamics (point attractor) by Marcial Losada
> Reprinted from Mathematical & Computer Modelling, Volume 30, The complex dynamics of high performance teams, pp. 179-192, 1999, with permission from Elsevier, license 1793240718833

Fig. 2-5B

Medium performance business team dynamics (mixed limit cycle and chaotic attractor) by Marcial Losada Reprinted from Mathematical & Computer Modelling, Volume 30, The complex dynamics of high performance teams, pp. 179-192, 1999, with permission from Elsevier, license 1793240718833

Fig. 2-5C

High performance business team dynamics (full Lorenz "butterfly" chaotic attractor) by Marcial Losada Reprinted from Mathematical & Computer Modelling, Volume 30, The complex dynamics of high performance teams, pp. 179-192, 1999, with permission from Elsevier, license 1793240718833

Fig. 2-6

Exploring Nature by Maartje van Caspel www.istockphoto.com, 676021, used with license.

Fig. 3-1

Fog in forest by Sergei Sverdelov www.istockphoto.com, 3893214, used with license.

Fig. 3-2

Inside the box 2 by Webking www.istockphoto.com, 492039, used with license.

Fig. 4-1

Sign- green glow opposite ways by Masterpiece
www.dreamstime.com, 258907, used with license.

Fig. 5-1

Evening prayer by Debi Bishop
www.istockphoto.com, 223837, used with license.

Fig. 6-1

Home improvement – your home is ready by Vasko
Miokovic
www.istockphoto.com, 422904, used with license.

Fig. 7-1

Blue curtain with path by Joshua Blake
www.istockphoto.com, 282832, used with license.

Fig. 7-2

Ruby red slippers by Mike Sonnenberg
www.istockphoto.com, 2515098, used with license.

Fig. E-1

Footprints in the sand at the beach by Brent Melton
www.istockphoto.com, 3017467, used with license.

About the Author

Iris R. Bell, MD PhD has been a researcher in areas related to complementary and alternative medicine for most of the past 30 years. She graduated magna cum laude in biology from Harvard University and then received her PhD in 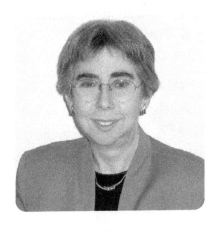 Neuro- and Biobehavioral Sciences (studying diet and sleep) and MD from Stanford University. Her psychiatry internship and residency were at the University of California – San Francisco, and she is Board certified in Psychiatry with Added Qualification in Geriatric Psychiatry. She is licensed to practice conventional medicine in Arizona and California. She is also nationally certified in biofeedback, a fellow of the American College of

Nutrition, and a licensed physician in homeopathy/integrative medicine in Arizona. She has served on the faculties of Harvard Medical School, University of California – San Francisco, and the University of Arizona.

She has published over 100 professional papers and a dozen book chapters on her clinical research in these areas. Her previous books range from the serious to the humorously fretful. She is the author of *Clinical Ecology: A New Medical Approach to Environmental Illness*, as well as two recent award-winning humor/inspiration books for people and pets with anxiety and worry, *Chew on Things – It Helps You Think: Words of Wisdom from a Worried Canine* and the *Chew on Things Workbook for Fellow Worriers*.

Her current research focuses on the relationship between complex systems and network science and philosophical bases of leading complementary and alternative medicine systems of care. She was chosen as one of the Best Doctors in the Pacific region of the US in 1996 and in the US in 1998. She is now a full-time researcher, educator, and writer.

She has also been a patient since her late teens, experiencing chronic health challenges that have ranged from migraine headaches to Type I diabetes mellitus and arthritis over the years. She has seen and experienced the good, the bad, and the ugly from both conventional and CAM treatments. For her tools as a patient, she has used an insulin pump, occasional other conventional medications, vitamin and mineral supplements, guided imagery, journaling, classical homeopathy, five-element acupuncture, osteopathy, naturopathy, Trager massage, subtle energy healing, and chiropractic.

Some treatments from both worlds have been helpful, and others have been harmful to her. Some practitioners from both conventional and CAM worlds have been supportive healers at critical points along the way, and some have been insensitive and out of touch. Certain tools have given her a major boost, others some benefit, and still others no help or even temporary setbacks. She knows that there is no single, perfect, or right answer for everyone with a chronic illness. Nonetheless, there are answers. Good answers.

She dedicates this book to people who find themselves with a chronic illness and are at the start of their own difficult journey home to themselves and to better health. This is a learning experience for us all.

http://www.GettingWhole.com

email ibell@GettingWhole.com

SPECIAL BONUS OFFER!
$97.00 worth of free bonus gifts

To thank you for taking action toward your own healing journey, three additional bonus gifts are waiting for you. The gifts are yours free as a reader of *Getting Whole, Getting Well*.

All you have to do to get your bonus gifts is visit our special website at: www.GettingWholeBonus.com, and the gifts are yours for immediate download and use.

Here's what you'll get:

- Your personal copy of *The Getting Whole, Getting Well Workbook*, ready for you to fill in your own thoughts, ideas, and imagery as you read the main book.

- A tips booklet on current choices from the best alternative medicine for preventing and treating the common cold and flu for yourself and your family.

- Dr. Bell's audio program (mp3 format), revealing the latest big picture healing tips, including additional practical ideas for finding your way to the holistic healing you need

Ready to get your free bonus gifts?

Come visit us at:

www.GettingWholeBonus.com

Join Our Community of People on their Healing Journey

Please follow the latest developments and share your ideas, thoughts, and comments in the world of personalized holistic healing at Dr. Bell's informative and thought-provoking blog:

http://www.HolisticMedicineTips.com

For readers who want to learn even more up-to-date exclusive information and enjoy in-depth discussions with other informed readers as part of a special community, participate in our online, members-only forum at:

http://www.HolisticMedicineTips.com/Members

Membership benefits include monthly live chats and teleseminars with Dr. Bell.

The first 100 readers of this book who sign up as charter members will receive a monthly 50% discount. All members will receive bonus discounts for purchases of additional books, CDs, and other products.

www.HolisticMedicineTips.com/Members
Enter discount coupon code: **GWGW**